Physiology and Pharmacology of the Heart

Physiology and Pharmacology of the Heart

Hilary Brown MA DPhil (Oxon)
University Research Lecturer
University Laboratory of Physiology
University of Oxford

Roland Kozlowski BSc (Bath), PhD (Cantab), MA (Oxon)
British Heart Foundation Lecturer
University Department of Pharmacology
University of Oxford

with clinical contributions by **Patrick Davey** MA (Oxon) MRCP

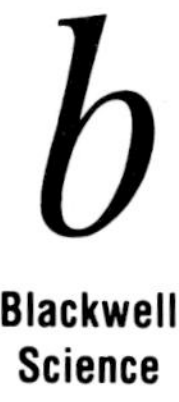

Blackwell
Science

Editorial Offices:
Osney Mead, Oxford OX2 0EL
25 John Street, London WC1N 2BL
23 Ainslie Place, Edinburgh EH3 6AJ
350 Main Street, Malden
MA 02148-5018, USA
54 University Street, Carlton
Victoria 3053, Australia

Other Editorial Offices:
Blackwell Wissenschafts-Verlag GmbH
Kurfürstendamm 57
10707 Berlin, Germany

Zehetnergasse 6
A-1140 Wien
Austria

First published 1997

Set by Excel Typesetters Co., Hong Kong
Printed and bound in Great Britain
at the University Press, Cambridge

Cover photograph Science Photo Library

DISTRIBUTORS

Marston Book Services Ltd
PO Box 269
Abingdon
Oxon OX14 4YN
(*Orders*: Tel: 01235 465500
Fax: 01235 465555)

USA
Blackwell Science, Inc.
Commerce Place
350 Main Street
Malden, MA 02148-5018
(*Orders*: Tel: 800 759-6102
617 388-8250
Fax: 617 388-8255)

Canada
Copp Clark Professional
200 Adelaide Street, West, 3rd Floor
Toronto, Ontario M5H 1W7
(*Orders*: Tel: 416 597-1616
800 815-9417
Fax: 416 597-1617)

Australia
Blackwell Science Pty Ltd
54 University Street
Carlton, Victoria 3053
(*Orders*: Tel: 3 9347 0300
Fax: 3 9347 5001)

A catalogue record for this title
is available from the British Library

ISBN 0-86542-722-4 (BSL)
0-86542-701-1 (IE)

Library of Congress
Cataloging-in-publication Data

Brown, Hilary, D.Phil.
Physiology and pharmacology of the heart
Hilary Brown and Roland Kozlowski
with clinical contributions by Patrick Davey.
p. cm.
Includes bibliographical references
and index
ISBN 0-86542-722-4
1. Heart—Physiology.
2. Heart—Effect of drugs on.
3. Cardiovascular agents.
4. Heart—Pathophysiology.
I. Kozlowski, Roland. II. Davey, Patrick.
III. Title. [DNLM: 1. Heart—physiology.
2. Heart Diseases—drug therapy.
3. Heart Diseases—physiopathology.
4. Cardiovascular Agents—therapeutic use.
WG 202 B878p 1996]
QP111.4.B76 1996
612.1′7—dc20
DNLM/DLC
for Library of Congress

96-18670
CIP

0 | Contents

Preface vii

Acknowledgements ix

Introduction: the work of the heart xi

1 Functional anatomy of the heart 1

2 Mechanical events during the cardiac cycle 7

3 The excitatory pathway 11

4 Cardiac cellular electrophysiology: ventricle and atrium 15

5 Cardiac cellular electrophysiology: pacemaking and conducting tissue 23

6 The electrocardiogram 31

7 Arrhythmias: electrophysiological basis 37

8 Antiarrhythmic drugs 43

9 Arrhythmias: clinical considerations 53

10 Excitation–contraction coupling and mechanoelectrical feedback 61

11 Functional aspects of cardiac muscle contraction 67

12 The nervous control of heart rate and force 71

13 Measurement of cardiac output 79

14 The cardiac environment: effects of altered ion concentrations on the heart 81

15 Coronary flow and coronary thrombosis 85

16 Drugs used to treat ischaemic heart disease 91

17 Cardiac failure 99

18 Drugs used for cardiac failure 103

19 Molecular biology of cardiac ion channels 109

20 Growing points in cardiac research 117

Further reading 121

Index 123

0 | Preface

We have written this book for those who are looking for a thorough background to their study of the heart. We have tried not to assume prior knowledge beyond A-level science and have aimed to take readers up to the stage at which they will start on original papers for themselves. Thus, while this is a textbook rather than a specialist research text, we have tried throughout to give glimpses of the most active research areas and of up-to-date clinical methods and treatment. The inclusion of clinical material will, we hope, be helpful to medical students in their beginning years whose courses are now integrated. We hope it will also prove interesting and useful to undergraduates studying physiology and other sciences related to medicine, to clinical medical students, to clinicians at various stages of their careers and in various specialties and to research workers moving into the field of heart research from other disciplines. We have not included detailed references but have listed some sources of further reading at the end of the book (p. 121).

Outline of this book

The anatomy of the heart is described in Chapter 1, which includes a brief account of the fetal circulation, the changes that occur at birth and the commonest congenital malformations of the heart. The mechanical events in the normal heart beat cycle are outlined in Chapter 2. Chapters 3–9 deal with the electrical excitatory system of the heart from membrane currents to arrhythmias and their treatment. Excitation-contraction coupling is the subject of Chapter 10 and mechanical properties of cardiac muscle and the influence of the nervous system on both these and on heart rate are considered in Chapters 11 and 12. Measurement of cardiac output and the effect of altered ion concentrations on the heart form the subjects of Chapters 13 and 14. The coronary circulation is described in Chapter 15, which goes on to consider the occurrence and treatment of ischaemic heart disease, the drugs for which are described in Chapter 16. Chapters 17 and 18 describe cardiac failure and its therapy. The molecular biology of cardiac ion channels forms the subject of Chapter 19 and a final brief chapter (Chapter 20) considers future perspectives in cardiac research and in the therapy of cardiac disease.

Hilary Brown
Roland Kozlowski

Acknowledgements

We should like to thank most warmly the following people who have read some or all of the manuscript and made helpful suggestions: Drs Michael Brown, Peter Kohl, David Paterson, Chris Plummer, Siân Rees, Martin Schuster Bruce, Professor David Eisner and Claire Sears. They are not, however, in any way to blame for any deficiencies of content or style which remain; those are entirely our responsibility.

We are also very grateful to the artist, David Gardner, for his work on the illustrations and to Andrew Robinson, Julie Elliott and the staff of Blackwell Science for continuing to remind us how slowly we were proceeding and for helping us at every stage of this book's production.

Hilary Brown
Roland Kozlowski
Patrick Davey

0 | Introduction: the work of the heart

The vast scale of the task the heart performs during a human lifetime is illustrated in the accompanying figure (Fig. 1). This diagram was prepared for a Japanese audience, so it uses as its unit the work done in raising an elephant up Mount Fuji. In a lifetime, the heart does work equivalent to raising 16 elephants such a height (3776 m): an impressive 240 million kg-m. In terms of fluid pumped, as the illustration also indicates, it empties 500 swimming pools.

The heart's performance is all the more amazing if one considers how rhythmic beating is maintained without failure or fatigue and with never more than a few hundred milliseconds' interval between beats. As important as the inbuilt rhythmicity are those mechanisms which allow recovery of both the electrical and contractile systems between each beat.

The normal adult human heart rate at rest is about 70 beats/min but it can rise in exercise to 200 beats/min. The volume of blood ejected per beat is called the stroke volume and in normal adults this is 90 ml at rest, rising to 140 ml in exercise. The product of stroke volume and heart rate gives the cardiac output: 6.5 l/min in the normal adult at rest, rising to 28 l/min in exercise. The figures given are for healthy young males; all these values vary with age and with fitness.

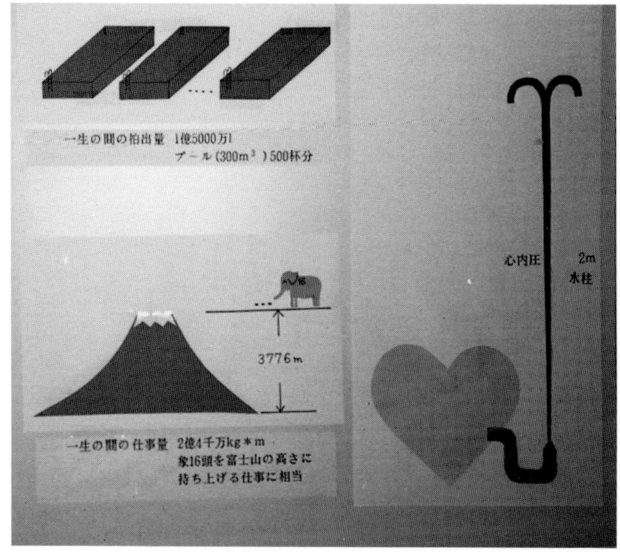

Figure 1
This poster was made for an 'open day' at a Japanese laboratory. The work accomplished by the heart during a human lifetime is comparable to that of raising 16 elephants the height of Mount Fuji and the amount of blood pumped is the equivalent of emptying 500 swimming pools. (Courtesy of Dr M. Kameyama.)

1 Functional anatomy of the heart

1.1 Introduction

The heart is a synchronized double pump, moving the blood sequentially around the pulmonary circulation (right side of the heart) and the systemic circulation (left side of the heart), as shown in Fig. 1.1. (For a schematic view of the adult circulation see Fig. 1.4b.) The wall thickness of each heart chamber is related to its function: the atria, within which only low pressures are developed, are relatively thin-walled. The left ventricle, which is the pump for the high-pressure systemic circulation, has a much thicker wall than the right ventricle, which has only to develop the lower pressures needed to pump blood through the pulmonary circulation.

1.2 Heart valves

The correct functioning of the heart depends on the efficiency of the valves separating the chambers, as would be the case for any pump. The valves can be seen in Fig. 1.1. Between atria and ventricles are the atrioventricular (AV) valves, which open to allow blood to flow into the ventricles during diastole (relaxation) and close during ventricular systole (contraction). These have descriptive names: the mitral valve (with paired cusps) on the left of the heart and the tricuspid valve on the right. On the ventricular sides of all the AV valves are ligaments called chordae tendinae, attached to the ventricular walls by projections known as papillary muscles.

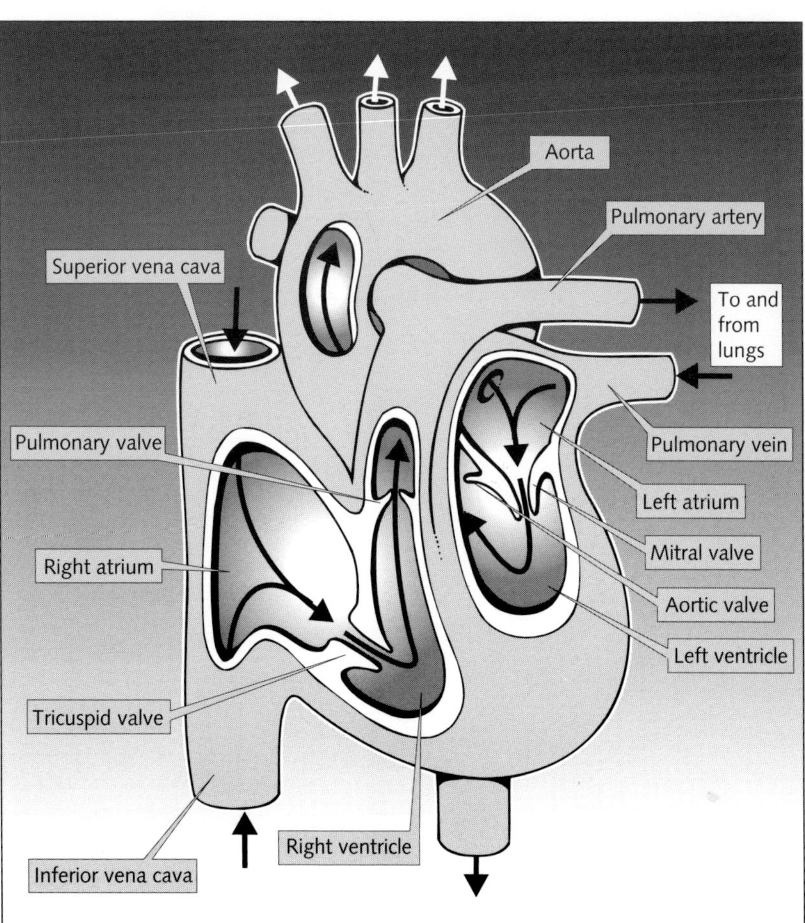

Figure 1.1
The heart and great vessels cut open longitudinally to show their structure and the direction of blood flow within them.

These prevent eversion of the closed valves when pressure rises during ventricular systole.

Between the ventricles and the aorta or pulmonary artery are the semilunar valves. Figure 1.2 shows an opened aorta to demonstrate the semilunar valves more clearly. In both the aorta and the pulmonary artery they consist of three cup-like cusps which open during ventricular systole and snap shut as ventricular pressure falls again.

1.3 Coronary vessels

Behind two of the three cusps of the aortic semilunar valves are located the orifices of the right and left coronary arteries. These can be seen in Fig. 1.2 and the arrangement is also shown in the inset. Coronary flow accounts for 5% of total cardiac output under resting conditions, rising to 8% in exercise. The delivery of this blood to ventricular muscle presents special problems because the contraction of the ventricular muscle itself impedes the blood flow in the coronary vessels. Most of this occurs, therefore, during diastole. The topic is considered in detail in Chapter 15. Here, it is sufficient to remember that unimpeded coronary flow is crucial for efficient cardiac function. Figure 1.3 illustrates the arrangement and profusion of the coronary vessels. Most of the coronary blood drains back into the heart through the coronary sinus which opens into the right atrium, but a small proportion of it flows directly into the ventricles through the anterior coronary and the Thebesian veins.

1.4 Circulatory changes at birth

1.4.1 The fetal circulation

During fetal life, as shown in Fig. 1.4, the circulation is arranged so it pumps a large quantity of blood through the placenta but little through the unexpanded lungs or through the liver, which is only partially functional.

The main differences from the adult circulation are:

- Oxygenated blood returning from the placenta through

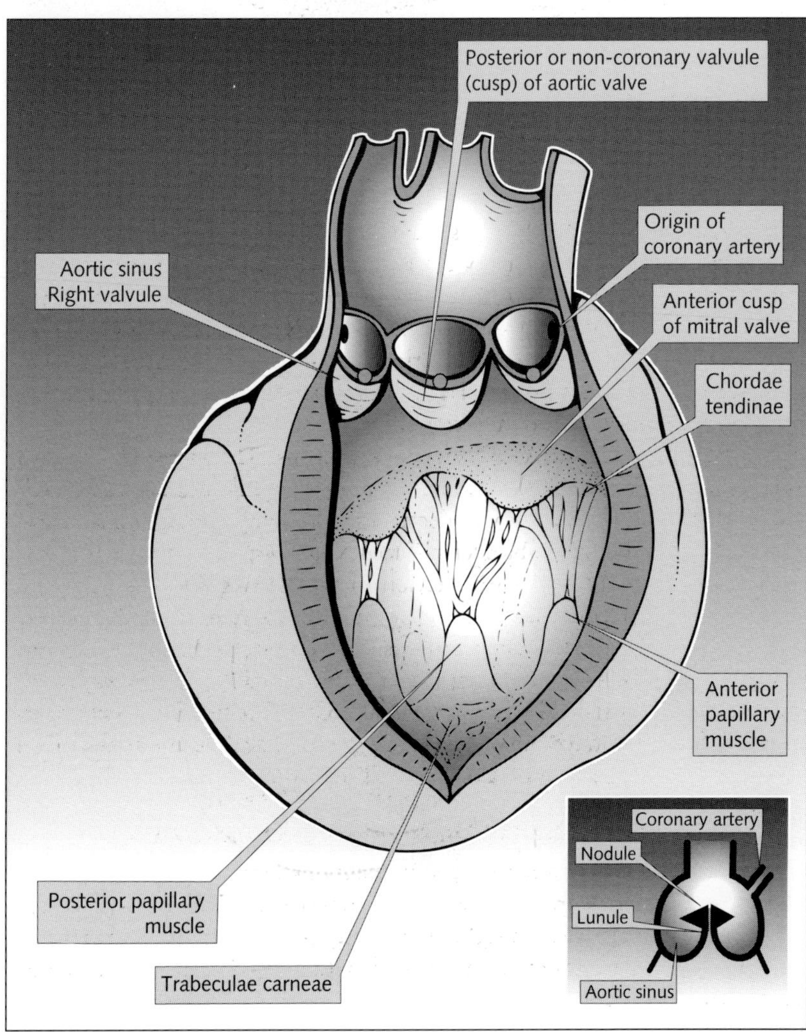

Figure 1.2
View of the left ventricle and aorta opened up to show more detail of the valves. The chordae tendinae (ligaments) and papillary muscles attach the atrioventricular (AV) valves firmly to the ventricle wall. Behind two of the cusps of the aortic semilunar valve are the openings of the coronary arteries (see inset).

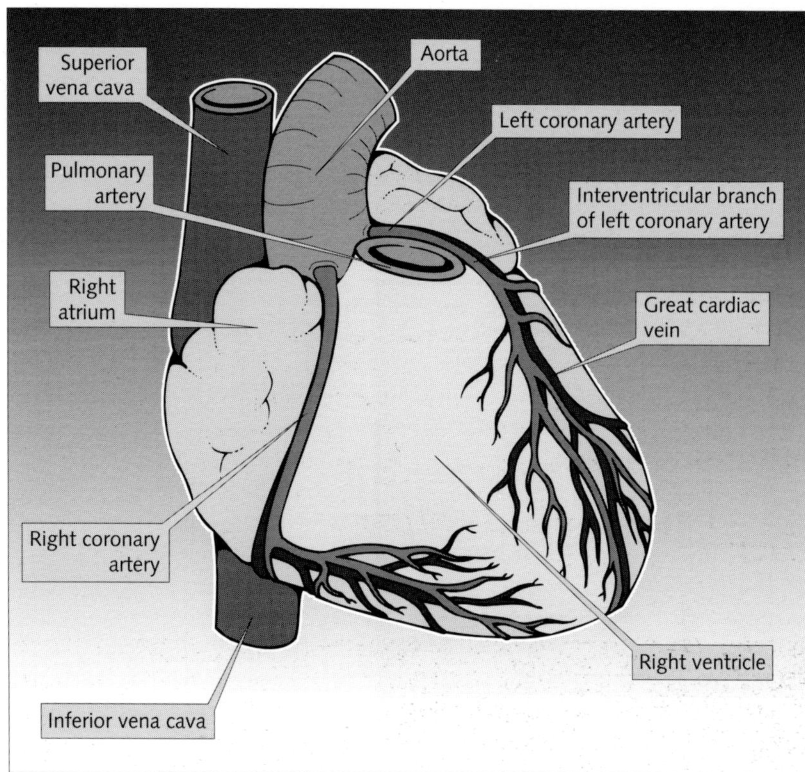

Figure 1.3
The coronary vessels.

the umbilical vein mostly bypasses the liver, enters the right atrium and passes directly through the foramen ovale to the left atrium. From the left ventricle it is pumped mainly to the head and forelimbs.

• The blood from the superior vena cava (mostly deoxygenated blood from the head region) passes downwards through the right atrium into the right ventricle and is pumped into the pulmonary artery where most of it passes through the ductus arteriosus into the aorta and thence through the umbilical arteries to the placenta for reoxygenation.

1.4.2 Circulatory changes at birth

At birth two primary changes occur in the circulation:

1 Loss of the large blood flow through the placenta approximately doubles the systemic vascular resistance, increasing the aortic pressure and the pressures in left atrium and left ventricle.

2 Expansion of the lungs removes both the compression of the pulmonary blood vessels and their hypoxia-induced vasoconstriction, resulting in a fivefold decrease in pulmonary vascular resistance. This reduces pulmonary arterial pressure and right ventricular and right atrial pressures.

These alterations in pressure cause:

3 Closure of the foramen ovale. As blood now tends to flow from the left to right atrium, rather than the other way as during fetal life, a small valve that lies over the foramen ovale on the left side of the atrial septum closes over the opening, preventing further flow. The closure becomes permanent within a few months in two-thirds of all people and in most others there is a functional closure since left atrial pressure remains 2–4 mmHg greater than the right atrial pressure, keeping the valve closed.

4 Closure of the ductus arteriosus. The increased systemic resistance elevates aortic pressure while the decreased pulmonary resistance decreases pulmonary arterial pressure. So, after birth, blood tends to flow through the ductus arteriosus in the opposite direction to that during fetal life (i.e. now from the aorta into the pulmonary artery). Within a few hours the ductus arteriosus constricts, probably in response to the greater oxygenation of the blood flowing through it. In most babies, the closure becomes functionally complete in 1–8 days and fibrous tissue grows to occlude the lumen of the ductus within a few months of birth.

1.5 Congenital malformations of the heart

1.5.1 Types of congenital malformation

There are three major types of congenital abnormality of the heart: left-to-right shunts, right-to-left shunts and stenosis (narrowing) of a channel within the heart or in a major vessel.

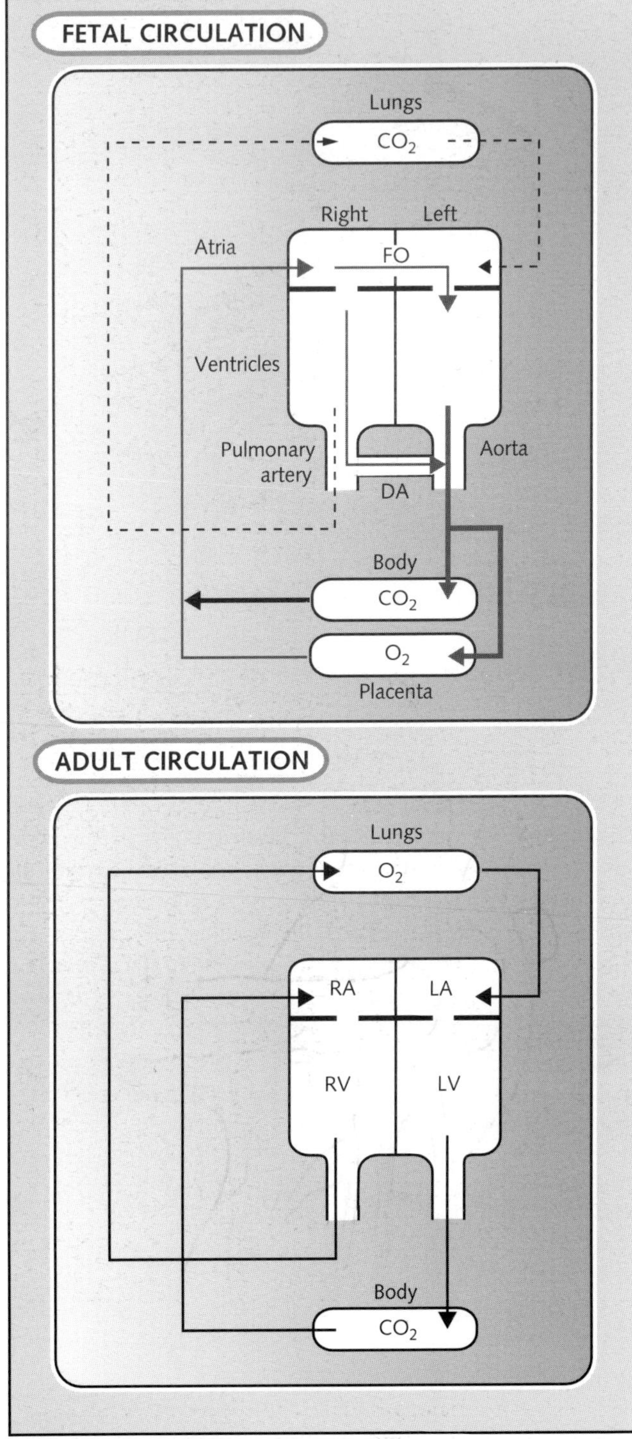

Figure 1.4
Schematic representation of the fetal circulation as compared with the adult circulation. In the fetus, relatively little blood goes to the lungs (dashed line) compared with that passing through the placenta, where oxygenation occurs. A considerable amount of blood passes from the right to the left atrium through the foramen ovale (FO) and from the pulmonary artery to the aorta through the ductus arteriosus (DA).

1.5.2 Left-to right shunts

These allow blood to flow from the left side of the heart or from the aorta to the right side of the heart or the pulmonary artery, thus bypassing the systemic circulation.

Patent ductus arteriosus is an example of a left-to-right shunt which occurs in 1 in 5500 babies when the ductus fails to close. It causes little trouble in the early months of life, but as the child grows older the difference in pressure between the aorta and the pulmonary artery increases and with it, the backward flow of blood from aorta to pulmonary artery. There is a huge extra flow of blood through the lungs and the output of the left ventricle may be two to three times normal, so that during exercise patients are unable to increase blood flow further and they feel weak, or may faint on attempting even moderate exercise. The heart hypertrophies: the left ventricle because of the extra work it must perform and the right ventricle because of increased pulmonary flow and consequent increased pressure within and sclerosis of the pulmonary blood vessels.

Patent ductus arteriosus is diagnosed from the poor response to exercise referred to above, together with hypertrophy of the heart, especially of the right ventricle, and a special type of heart murmur, the 'machinery murmur' which arises from flow through the patent ductus which is most intense during systole. Surgical correction (ligation of the patent ductus arteriosus) is simple; if uncorrected, patients die from heart failure between 20 and 40 years old.

Other left-to-right shunts with basically similar consequences are interventricular and interatrial septal defects; the latter occur most commonly when the foramen ovale does not close properly at birth. The circulation through the heart when there is atrial septal defect is shown in Fig. 1.5b.

1.5.3 Right-to-left shunts

These allow blood to flow from the right side of the heart or pulmonary artery directly into the left side of the heart or the aorta, thus bypassing the lungs.

An example of this type of shunt is the tetralogy of Fallot (Fig. 1.5c) in which four abnormalities occur together:

1 The aorta originates wholly or in part from the right ventricle rather than the left.

2 The pulmonary artery is stenosed so that less blood than normal passes from the right ventricle to the lungs; instead it goes into the aorta.

3 Blood from the right ventricle flows through a ventricular septal defect into the left ventricle.

4 The right ventricle, which pumps large amounts of blood into the aorta, against high pressure, becomes enlarged.

A feature of this condition is cyanosis, caused by both the reduced flow through the lungs because of the pulmonary stenosis and by the aorta's receiving blood from the right as well as from the left ventricle. Fallot's tetralogy is the most

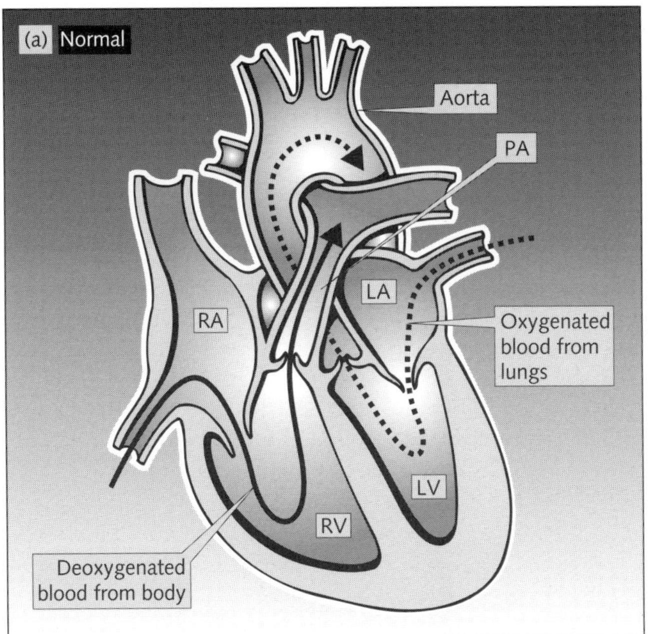

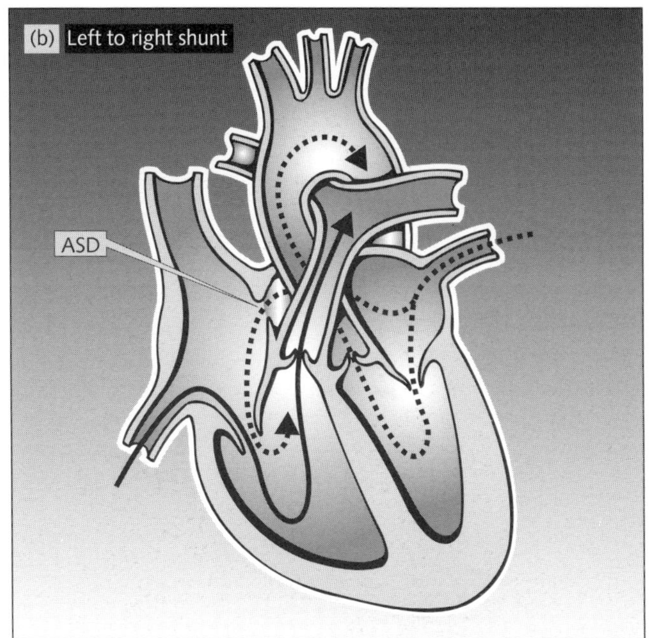

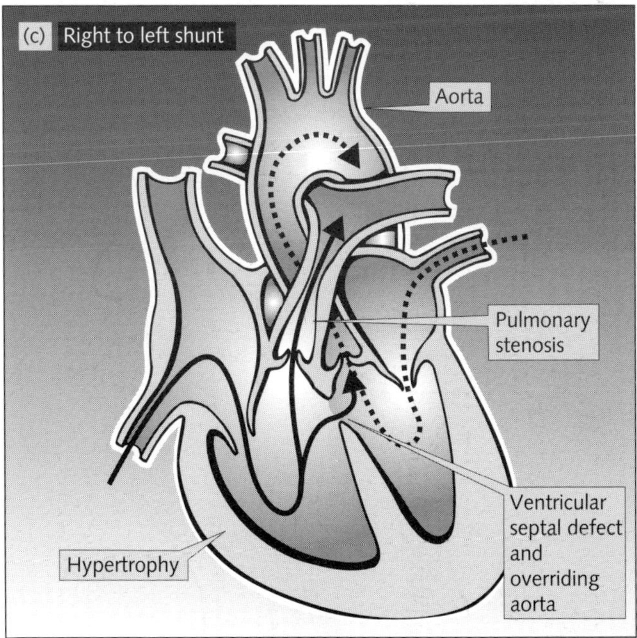

Figure 1.5
Congenital malformations of the heart. Diagrammatic sections through the heart and great vessels showing normal circulation (a), atrial septal defect, an example of left-to-right shunt (b) and in (c), the tetralogy of Fallot an example of right-to-left shunt; see text. RA, LA, right and left atria; RV, LV, right and left ventricles; PA, pulmonary artery; ASD, atrial septal defect. Flow of deoxygenated blood (solid lines); flow of oxygenated blood (dotted lines).

common cause of 'blue' babies; the reduced oxygenation of arterial blood is a diagnostic feature, along with enlarged right ventricle (with high systolic pressures recorded within it by catheter). The anatomical abnormalities can be seen in echocardiographs.

1.5.4 Stenosis

Stenosis of a channel constricts blood flow at some point in the heart or in a major vessel near the heart. Points at which congenital stenosis commonly occur are in the aorta (particularly at the level of the aortic valves) and in the lungs (pulmonary stenosis) leading to enlargement of the left and of the right ventricle, respectively, and to characteristic heart murmurs. The constriction can usually be successfully enlarged surgically.

2 Mechanical events during the cardiac cycle

2.1 The changes in pressure during a heart beat

Figure 2.1 shows the pressure changes in the chambers of the heart and in the aorta during the cardiac cycle, together with the alterations in ventricular volume. The following description is of events occurring in the left side of the heart; those in the right heart are similar but the pressures in the right chambers are much smaller, as shown in part (b) of Fig. 2.1. The timings given are those at a resting heart rate.

- A–B. During diastole, the mitral valves are open and blood flows from the pulmonary veins through the left atrium into the left ventricle.
- B–C. Contraction of the left atrium 'tops up' the blood already in the left ventricle, contributing 20% (at age 20) to 40% (at age 80) of left ventricular filling.
- C–D. As the ventricles begin to contract, the pressure in the left ventricle rapidly overtakes that in the left atrium so that the mitral valve closes. With both atrioventricular (AV) and semilunar (aortic) valves closed, the ventricle at first contracts with little or no volume change (isovolumetrically). Pressure within the ventricles increases rapidly.
- D. Pressure in the left ventricle exceeds that in the aorta so that the semilunar valve opens (point D) and about 90 ml of blood (the stroke volume) is ejected into the aorta, leaving about 50 ml within the left ventricle (the end-systolic volume).
- D–E. The volume of the ventricles rapidly diminishes. This is the period of so-called isotonic contraction of the ventricular muscle — shortening of the muscle with little further increase in tension.
- E–F. Aortic pressure declines from its peak as run-off from the aorta to the periphery exceeds ventricular output. Throughout ventricular systole the blood returning to the atria produces a progressive rise in atrial pressure. There is a suction effect caused by displacement of the AV border during ventricular contraction which assists blood to flow into the atria from the veins. When pressure in the left ventricle falls below that in the aorta, the aortic valve closes (point F). This point is considered the end of ventricular systole which has lasted 300 ms. Closure of the aortic valves causes a notch (the incisura or dichrotic notch) on the descending limb of the aortic pressure curve.
- F–G. A short period of isovolumetric relaxation while both semilunar AV valves are closed starts ventricular diastole (relaxation), which occupies the next 550 ms.
- G–A. When ventricular pressure falls below that in the atrium, the AV valves open (point G). It is now that the major part of ventricular filling occurs as venous blood which had continuously entered the atria during the previous ventricular systole is suddenly released into the ventricles by the opening of the AV valves. There is a sharp decrease in both atrial and ventricular pressures and a rapid increase in ventricular volume. This initial rapid filling phase is succeeded by the phase of slow filling (A–B) during which atrial and ventricular pressures rise again as venous blood continues to flow into them.

2.2 Pressure changes in the right heart

In part (b) of Fig. 2.1 the pressure changes in the chambers of the right side of the heart are shown. They follow the same general pattern as those in the left heart but they are much smaller. The volume changes are the same as those in the left heart, as Fig. 2.1 shows, since the two sides of the heart lie in series in the circulation and so must pump the same volumes of blood.

2.3 Monitoring the heart's performance

There are several important ways of monitoring the events in the cardiac cycle. These include echocardiography, electrocardiography, listening to the heart sounds, observing the venous pulse and catheterization.

2.3.1 The electrocardiogram

The electrocardiogram (ECG) is indicated at the bottom of Fig. 2.1. It will be explained in detail in Chapter 6.

2.3.2 Heart sounds

The heart sounds are also indicated in Fig. 2.1. They are traditionally those audible through a stethoscope, though more sophisticated amplifiers can now pick up additional sounds. The first heart sound occurs as the AV valves close and is normally the loudest. It is caused partly by vibrations of the AV valves on closure and of the adjacent cardiac wall and partly by turbulence of the blood. The second heart sound is heard when the semilunar (aortic and pulmonary) valves close. It is often split, especially during inspiration because the aortic valves close slightly before the pulmonary valves. A third heart sound, heard in early diastole, can be associated with

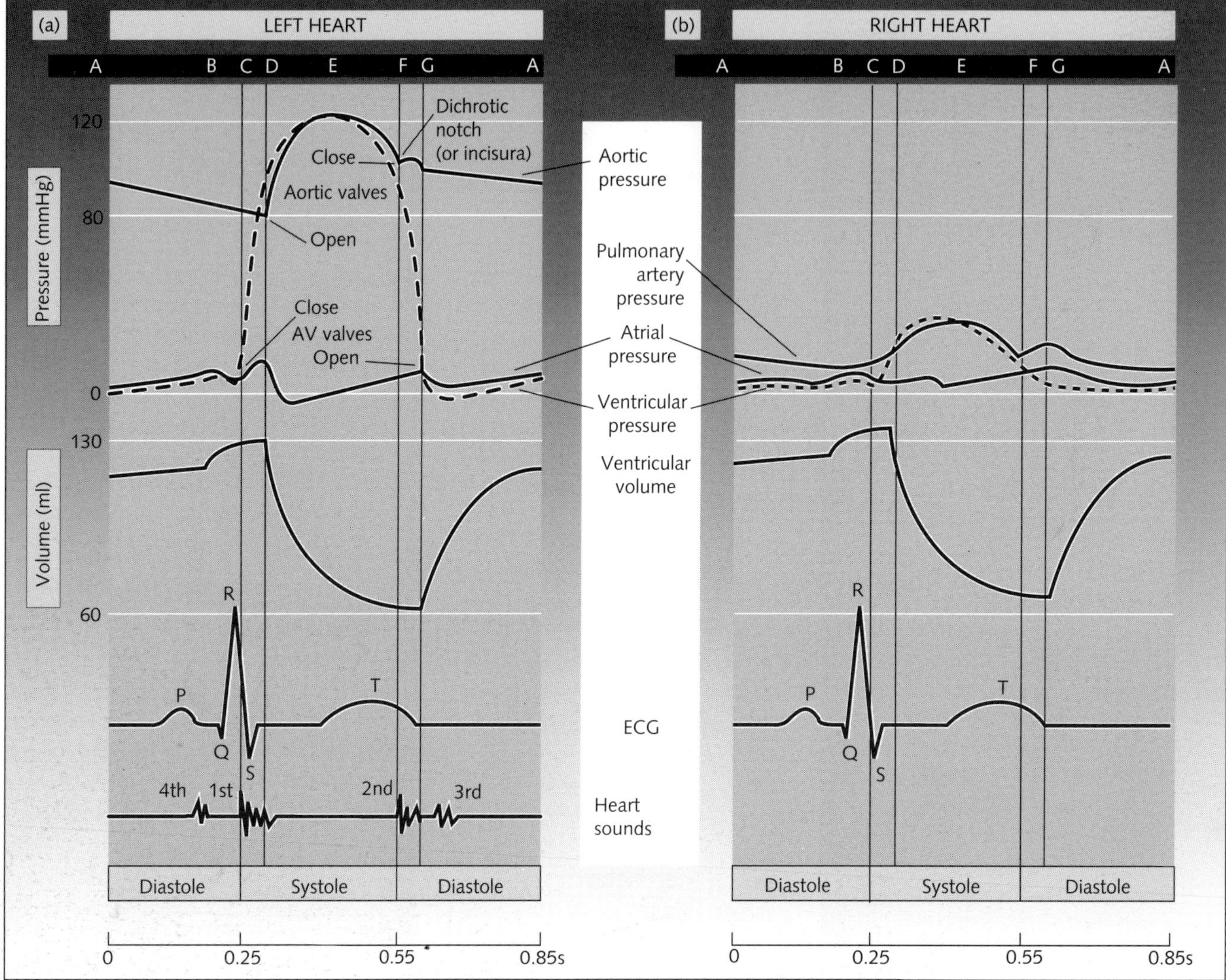

Figure 2.1
Pressure changes in the chambers of the left (a) and of the right (b) heart during a cardiac cycle and (below) changes in ventricular volume. The electrocardiogram (see Chapter 6) is also shown and the heart sounds are indicated. See text.

the rapid filling of the ventricles with blood that had accumulated in the atria, and a fourth heart sound occurs just before the first sound, associated with atrial systole. The third and fourth sounds are low pitched and difficult to hear.

Abnormal heart sounds may result from a variety of causes. If blood passes through a narrowed orifice or regurgitates back through an incompetent valve, its flow becomes turbulent and this may generate murmurs. Thus, malfunctions of the valves give characteristic murmurs.

Congenital cardiac abnormalities also give rise to abnormal heart sounds. Thus, when the ductus arteriosus remains patent instead of closing at birth (Chapter 1), a continuous murmur will be present throughout the cardiac cycle. If there is a congenital defect in the atrial septum, a systolic murmur can be heard, while a congenital interventricular connection will give a different form of systolic murmur.

2.3.3 The jugular venous pulse

The changes in pressure in the right atrium are transmitted into the large veins and can be seen as pulsations in the internal jugular vein in the neck. Jugular venous pressure (JVP) is compared in Fig. 2.2 with pressure changes in the right atrium and with those in the carotid artery. Each peak occurs a little later in the jugular vein than in the right atrium. There are three peaks in the JVP—the a, c and v waves:

- The a (atrial) wave occurs just after atrial contraction. It is

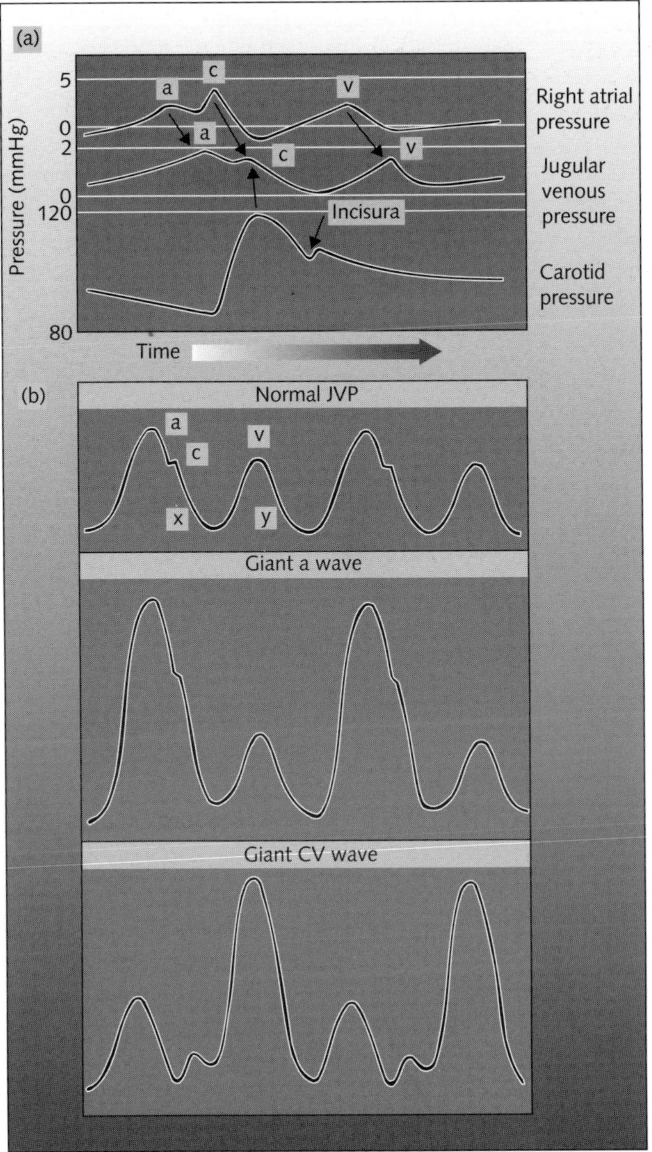

Figure 2.2
(a) Temporal relationships between the jugular venous pressure, right atrial pressure and carotid arterial pressure. (b) Two examples of abnormal jugular venous pressure traces are compared with a normal trace (top). In the normal trace, the so-called x and y descents are marked, after the c and v waves. The second trace shows giant 'a' waves which occur because of atrial contraction against a stenosed tricuspid valve. The giant 'cv' waves seen in the bottom trace occur when the right ventricular pressure is transmitted back to the right atrium through a regurgitant tricuspid valve. (Records in (b) courtesy of Dr C.J. Plummer, Freeman Hospital, Newcastle upon Tyne.)

augmented by damming of blood in the large veins as atrial contraction constricts the orifices of the venae cavae.

• The c (carotid) wave is a delayed reflection of the rise in atrial pressure when, as the ventricle contracts, the (tricuspid) AV valve bulges into the atrium. Added to this, the pressure pulse is transmitted from the adjacent carotid artery during peak systole, hence the term c wave.

• The third, v (venous), wave again occurs slightly later than the corresponding right atrial pressure peak which itself results from blood inflow from the venous system during the period when the AV valves are closed (i.e. during ventricular systole plus the phase of isometric relaxation).

The jugular pulse waves are influenced by intrathoracic pressure fluctuations associated with breathing but changes in the JVP can nevertheless indicate the presence of cardiac arrhythmias, valvular incompetence or rises in right atrial pressure. Two examples of abnormal JVP records are shown in Fig. 2.2b.

2.3.4 Echocardiography

Echocardiography is a non-invasive technique and is increasingly used to monitor cardiac performance. The reflections of ultrasound waves from different structures in the heart give

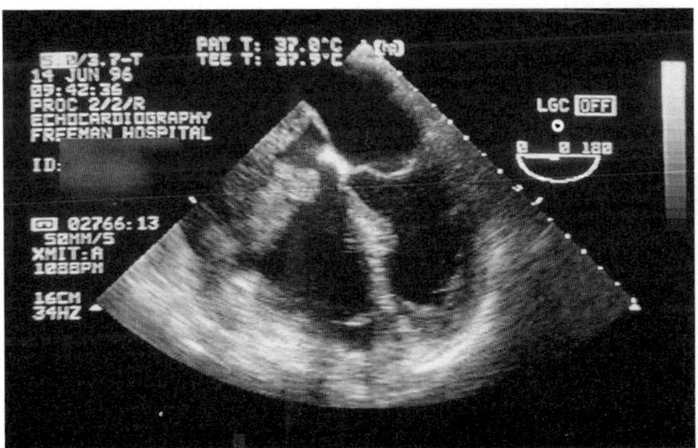

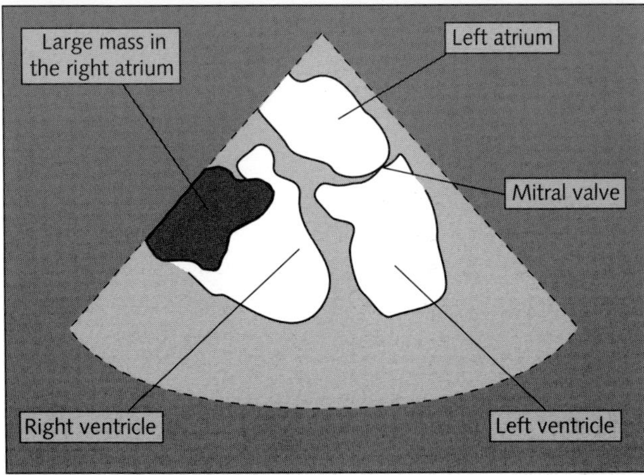

Figure 2.3
Transoesophageal echocardiograph showing a large mass in the right atrium. (Courtesy of Dr C.J. Plummer, Freeman Hospital, Newcastle upon Tyne.)

detailed images of both structures and their movements during the cardiac cycle.

• Two-dimensional echocardiography gives a fan-shaped image of a cross-section at a given plane; it can show all four chambers (Fig. 2.3).

• M-mode echocardiography gives pictures of structures in a single narrow beam below the transducer and can give a display of heart function thoughout the cardiac cycle showing, for example, the movements of the valves.

Doppler echocardiography is a refinement of this technique which gives additional information about blood flow.

2.3.5 Cardiac catheterization

This clinically very important technique involves introducing a catheter into the heart through an artery, for the left side of the heart, or through a vein, for the right side of the heart. The catheter is manipulated to the required site within the heart or great vessels using imaging and can be used to measure pressures, to sample blood and/or measure its oxygen saturation and to inject radiopaque material for the study of blood flow or of the anatomy of the heart and vessels. Catheters are also used in angioplasty where a balloon is inflated to widen a blocked coronary artery (see Chapter 15).

2.3.6 Nuclear cardiology

• Injected thallium-201 can be used to monitor myocardial perfusion and to detect focal ischaemia during exercise tests.

• Magnetic resonance imaging is rarely used clinically because of the cost and time needed to acquire an image (as much as 40 min) but it is useful for diagnosing pericardial disease.

3 The excitatory pathway

3.1 Intercellular connections

All cardiac muscle cells are electrically connected to one another by low-resistance connections so that the whole heart behaves electrically as if it were a single cell. Thus the electrical impulse, once initiated, spreads through the heart muscle in the same way as that in which a nerve impulse spreads along a nerve fibre. This is shown schematically in Fig. 3.1. The multiply folded boundaries between adjacent cells (the intercalated discs) form gap junctions over about 5% of their length, where the membranes of the cells come into very close apposition and contain a group of areas of high conductance called nexi (singular: nexus). This arrangement is shown at various magnifications in Fig. 3.2. Figure 3.3 shows gap junctions between ventricular cells under the electron microscope in both section and in surface view.

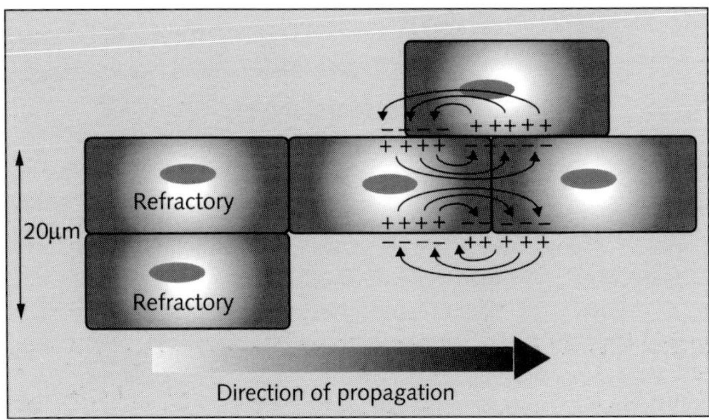

Figure 3.1
Spread of excitation through the cardiac syncytium. The small arrows indicate the flow of local currents ahead of the active region.

Figure 3.2
Junctional region between two cardiac myocytes at increasing magnifications. (b) corresponds to part of the electron micrograph shown in Fig. 3.3a. In (d) it can be seen that a single nexus is formed of two halves protruding into the cytoplasm of the cell and at the extracellular side each is linked tightly to the other half-channel that is its mirror image in the membrane of the neighbouring cell. Each half-channel, or connexon, is composed of six protein subunits (only 3 shown) arranged around a central fluid-filled pore of about 1.5 nm diameter, the region of high conductance.

3.2 The pacemaker region

The rhythm of the vertebrate heart is myogenic, that is, it originates in the heart muscle itself. When the heart is in the

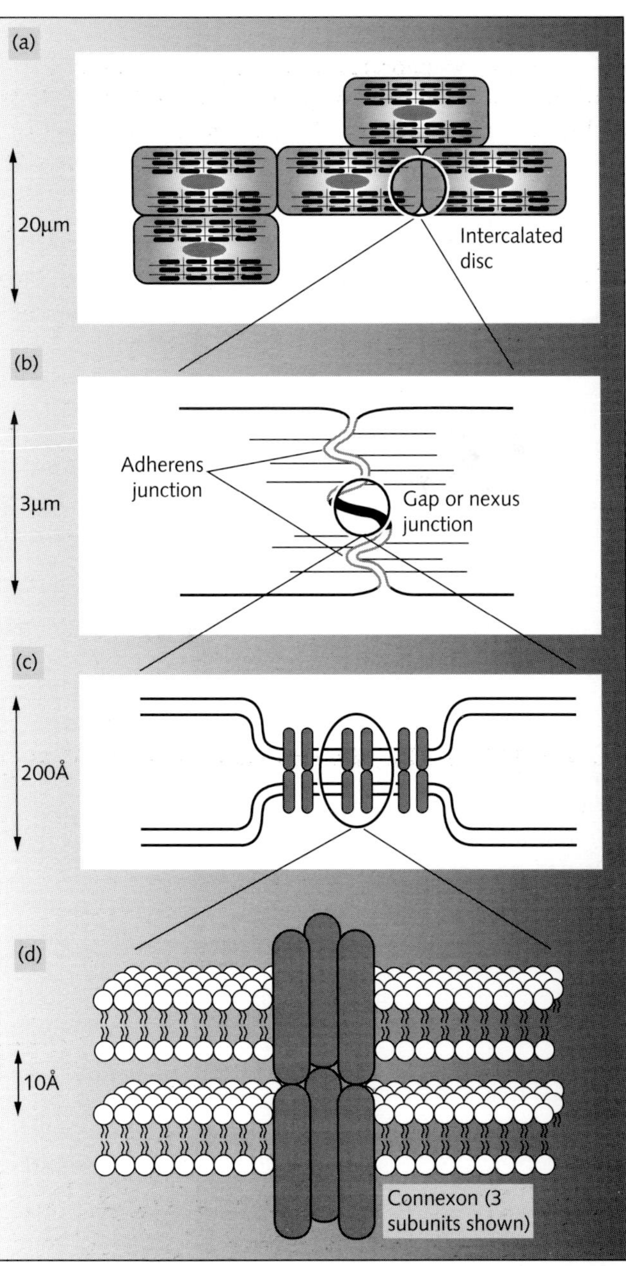

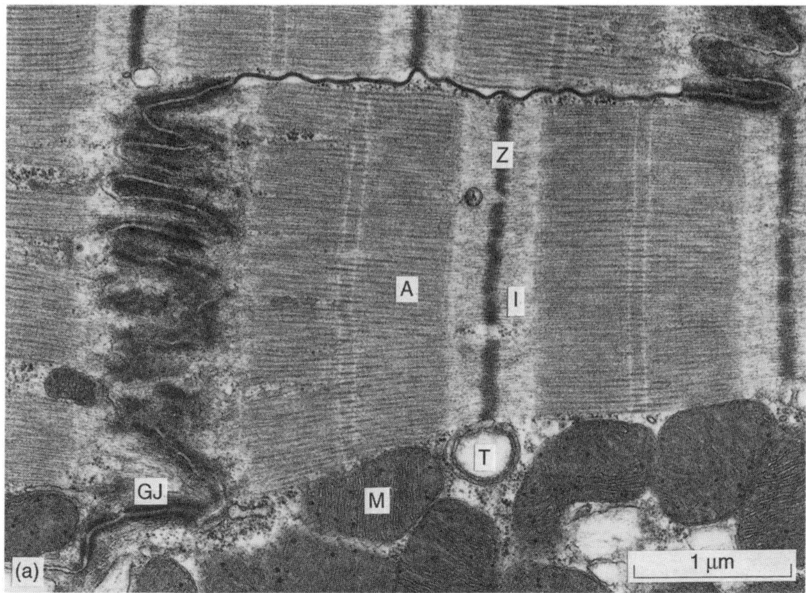

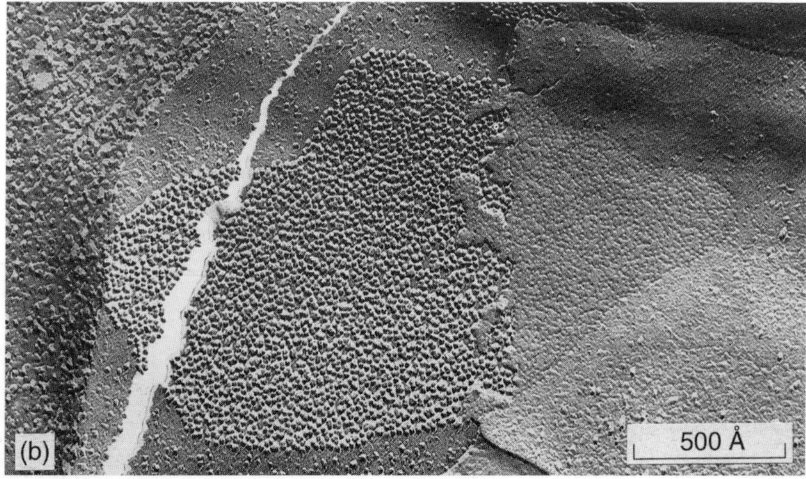

Figure 3.3
Electron micrograph of part of the folded junctional region (the intercalated disc) between two ventricular cells. Nexi can be seen at intervals. A freeze fracture surface view of a gap junction is shown in (b). (Courtesy of Dr N. Severs.) GJ, gap junction; A, I, A and I bands; Z, Z line; T, T-tubule; M, mitochondrion.

body this rhythm is influenced by nerves and by circulating hormones. William Harvey (1628) recognized that normally the beat was initiated in the right atrium and from there passed to the other heart chambers.

The pacemaker region of the mammalian heart, the sinoatrial (SA) node, was first described by Keith and Flack in 1907. Martin Flack was a medical student working during the summer in the histological laboratory that Professor (later Sir Arthur) Keith had set up in his vacation house in Kent. While Keith and his wife were out on a cycle ride one evening, Flack was looking at heart sections and came across a richly innervated region of small muscle cells in the wall of the right atrium between the entry points of the superior and inferior venae cavae, which looked very like the atrioventricular (AV) nodal tissue described a short time previously by the Japanese histologist, Tawara.

Later, Flack went on to show that the application of heat or cold to this area was particularly effective in influencing heart rhythm and soon it was demonstrated that this was also the region which showed 'initial negativity' (the first sign of electrical activity recorded externally) at each heart beat. More detail of the organization of the SA node and of its pacemaking role will be given in Chapter 5.

3.3 Conduction of excitation

In addition to the SA node where the excitatory impulses normally arise, there are other areas of cardiac muscle which have become specialized for autonomous excitation or for conduction. They can also provide subsidiary pacemakers should the primary pacemaker fail or conduction become blocked. Normally they will be driven by the impulses arriv-

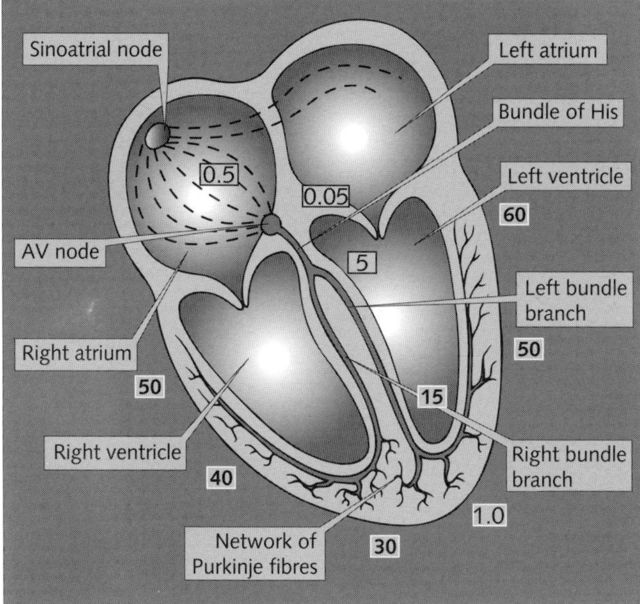

Figure 3.4
The timing, in milliseconds, of the spread of the excitatory impulse through the heart. Large figures: speed of impulse in m/s; small figures: time elapsed (in ms) for impulse to travel from AV node to various points of the ventricle. Note the delay of conduction within the AV node and rapid passage of excitation down the bundle of His (the Purkinje fibres) to all points of the ventricle.

ing from the SA node which has the highest intrinsic rate of firing.

The timing of the spread of the impulse from the SA node to the other regions of the heart is shown in Fig. 3.4. In round figures, the excitatory wavefront takes:

- 45 ms to emerge from the SA node.
- 40 ms to travel across the atria.
- At least 100 ms to go through the AV node.
- 30 ms to be conducted through the Purkinje system.
- 30 ms to travel throughout the ventricular muscle.

The delay in the AV node is functionally very important, for it allows time for atrial contraction to move blood into the ventricles before they receive the signal to contract. It is crucial, too, that all regions of the ventricular muscle should be excited as nearly synchronously as possible, so once through the AV node, the impulse is conducted very rapidly to all points of the ventricle by the Purkinje fibres—muscle fibres which have become specialized for rapid conduction, rather than for contraction, which they do only weakly. As indicated in Fig. 3.4, after it has left the AV node, the impulse travels very rapidly down the Purkinje fibres (here grouped together to form the bundle of His) which run in the interventricular septum and then up the inner surfaces of the ventricles. Thus excitation reaches all parts of the ventricular muscle within 30 ms, leading to a virtually synchronous contraction. The arrangement of the Purkinje fibres is very clearly seen in the preparation shown in Fig. 3.5, which was made by Sir Thomas Lewis, a leading cardiologist in the early part of this century, by injecting Indian ink into the bundle of His of a cow heart.

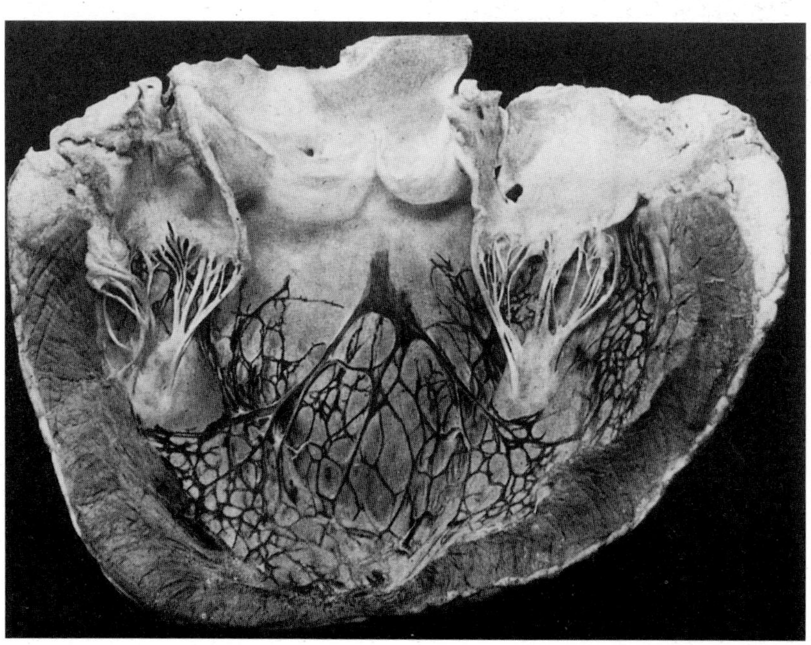

Figure 3.5
In this preparation of a cow's heart the network of Purkinje fibres of the left ventricle was injected with Indian ink and shows clearly against the inner surface of the opened left ventricle. (From Lewis, T. (1925) *Mechanism and Graphic Registration of the Heart Beat.* Shaw & Sons, London.)

4 Cardiac cellular electrophysiology: ventricle and atrium

4.1 Recording methods

The summated electrical activity of cardiac muscle can be recorded from the outside of the heart or even from the outside of the body as the electrical impulse sweeps across the membrane of every cardiac cell to trigger each heart beat. Such records comprise the electrocardiogram or ECG. In the last century ingenious experiments on 'animal electricity' had revealed some properties of the excitatory impulses. For example, Kolliker and Müller (1856) demonstrated that a frog's sciatic nerve laid across an active ventricle would be excited twice at each heart beat, indicating that the electrical event was much longer in cardiac muscle than in nerve. The development of the string galvanometer by Einthoven (1903) allowed the first clear records of the ECG to be made and the ECG was in routine diagnostic use by the 1920s. The ECG is considered in detail in Chapter 6.

Recording intracellular action potentials from cardiac muscle was not possible until the development in the 1950s of the glass microelectrode which could be inserted into individual cells without excessive damage to their membranes, but there were still many technical problems associated with obtaining stable records and with applying a voltage clamp to cardiac muscle. The electrical activity in heart as in other muscle and nerve cells is associated with the flow of ions across the cell membrane. To understand the ionic currents it is necessary to record the current flow at constant voltage—a technique known as voltage clamping.

Further problems arose from the arrangement of cardiac muscle in a three-dimensional network which made it hard to maintain a constant voltage across any reasonable length of membrane from a point source of control (the microelectrode). This problem was avoided by concentrating on Purkinje fibres where specialization for conduction has given larger cells grouped in fairly uniform cylinders to which the voltage clamp technique could more easily be applied.

Once the technique for isolating individual cardiac cells had been developed (from the late 1970s on), most of these problems could be overcome. The single cell can be voltage clamped either using a standard microelectrode which switches constantly and rapidly (at 3 Hz) between current and voltage recording (switch clamp) or by using a patch clamp electrode in the 'whole cell' mode (Fig. 4.1 and see Chapter 19 for an explanation of this technique). This latter method has the advantages that it can also be applied to the smaller cardiac cells of the sinoatrial (SA) and atrioventricular (AV) nodes, which are damaged by microelectrode penetration, and that it can be combined with introducing desired ions or indicators into the cell interior by perfusing them through the electrode. The opening and closing of single channels in the cell membrane can also be recorded from membrane patches in the cell-attached or detached modes (see Fig. 4.1e and Chapter 19), giving a new level of analysis of membrane excitability.

The excitement of being able to apply these new techniques to single cardiac cells should not obscure the fact that the cells are *single* and some properties of heart excitation such as conduction, fibrillation, heart block and so on can only be studied in groups of cells or, indeed, in whole hearts, either isolated and perfused or within the animal or patient.

Figure 4.1 summarizes the development of methods of recording electrical events from cardiac cells.

4.2 The ventricular cell

The nature of cellular electrical activity varies considerably from region to region of the heart. Before considering the special features of excitation in nodal and conducting tissue, we will focus on the ventricular myocyte, arguably the most important and certainly the most numerous of cardiac cells. The following account assumes that the reader is already familiar, at least in outline, with the mechanism of the resting and action potential of the nerve fibre.

It is appropriate to consider a single ventricular cell, such as is shown in Fig. 4.2. To obtain isolated cells, the heart of an experimental animal (usually a guinea-pig or rat) is back-perfused by the Langendorff method, that is, through a cannula placed in the aorta so that perfusion fluid is forced through the coronary arteries. The perfusion fluid used contains enzymes such as collagenase, which in the presence of very low (20–50 μmol/l), but not zero, calcium concentration will break the intercellular connections while leaving the cell membranes undamaged and able to withstand the return to normal calcium levels.

4.3 The ventricular action potential: general features

A typical action potential of a mammalian (guinea-pig) ventricular cell is shown in Fig. 4.3. The most striking difference between it and the action potential of a nerve fibre or that of a

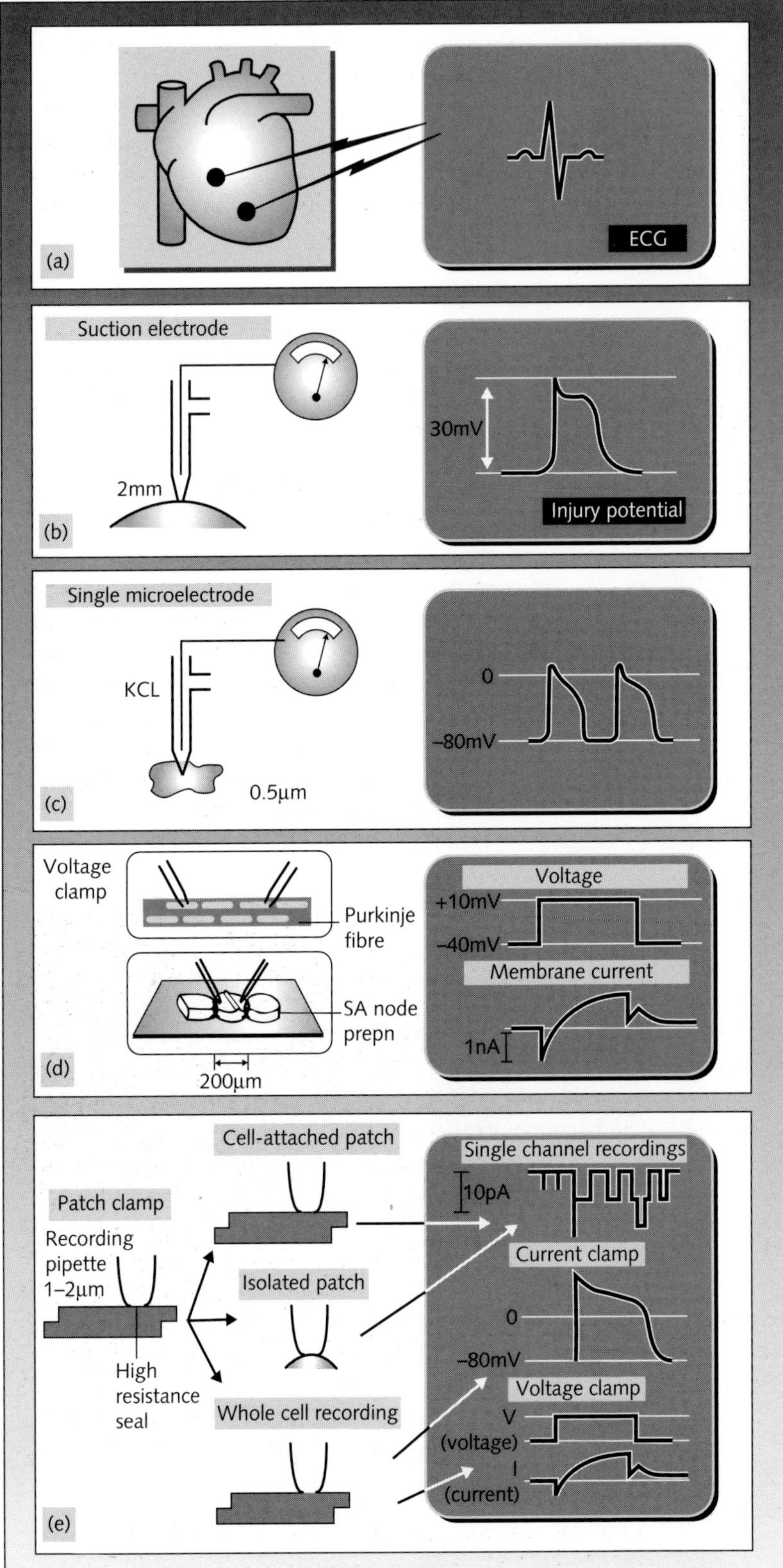

Figure 4.1
Methods of recording the electrical activity of cardiac muscle. (a) Surface recording of the electrocardiogram. (b) A suction electrode applied to the surface of the heart sucks up and injures a small amount of tissue thus gaining electrical access to the intracellular side of the muscle membranes. Injury potentials and monophasic action potentials can be recorded relative to another electrode on an uninjured part of the muscle. These are similar to resting potentials and action potentials but shortcircuiting means they are considerably smaller. (c) Glass microelectrodes (tip diameter 0.5 μm or less) pierce cell membranes without damaging them and allow electrical recording from many types of individual cardiac muscle cells. If the tissue is moving the microelectrodes can be made long and flexible or mounted on flexible wires. (d) Voltage clamp of multicellular preparations can be achieved in Purkinje fibres, or in small preparations of SA node ligated with fine thread, using two microelectrodes. (e) Once a high resistance seal has been made between a patch electrode and the membrane of an isolated cardiac muscle cell, various recording modes are possible: single channels can be recorded from cell-attached or isolated patches of membrane or the membrane patch within the pipette tip can be disrupted (or made permeable to small ions) for whole cell recording in current clamp or voltage clamp mode.

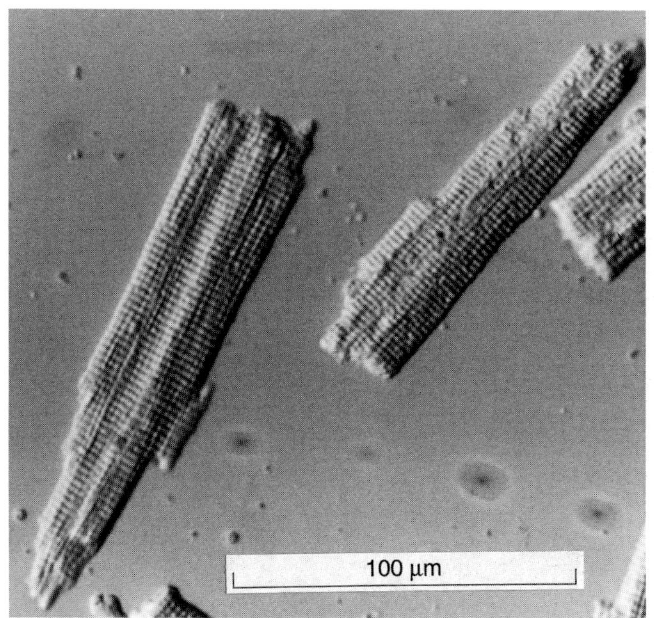

Figure 4.2
Freshly isolated ventricular cells from a guinea-pig. The isolation procedure consists of back-perfusion of the coronary circulation via the aorta with a solution containing enzymes such as collagenase which in the presence of very low calcium concentrations will break the intercellular attachments without harming the individual cells. (Courtesy of Dr Allan Levi.)

skeletal muscle cell is its far longer duration: 200–300 ms as compared to 1–5 ms. Like nerve or skeletal muscle, ventricular muscle has a negative resting potential (better called diastolic potential) of about −80 mV. After the initial upstroke the ventricular action potential has a prolonged plateau phase during which the potential within the cell stays at around 0 mV until, after 200–300 ms, repolarization occurs. Figure 4.3 shows the time relations between a ventricular action potential and the contraction it triggers.

4.4 Refractory period

Such a long action potential is associated with a very long refractory period, during which another stimulus cannot excite a response, which lasts almost as long as the action potential itself. Figure 4.4 shows the electrical responses when a ventricular cell is stimulated at different times in the cardiac cycle: the long absolute refractory period is followed by a relative refractory period during which smaller action potentials than normal are produced.

The adaptive nature of such an arrangement for a rhythmically beating system is illustrated in Fig. 4.4. This shows the effects on cardiac contraction of an applied stimulus given at different times during the cardiac cycle. The records are traces of the contractions of a frog's ventricle, but the same result could be obtained with a mammalian heart. During the first part of the cardiac cycle an applied stimulus has no effect. By the time in the cycle that the extra stimulus does produce an extra response, the ventricle is already relaxing after the normal contraction so that two independent contractions result. There can be no summation of responses (no tetanus) as there is in skeletal muscle. This is clearly important for the heart where regular independent beats are essential.

The long cardiac action potential is not just a trigger of the contractile response, as is the brief action potential of a skeletal muscle fibre, it can also itself modulate the strength of contraction, particularly when the amount of contributing inward calcium current varies.

4.5 Membrane currents underlying the ventricular action potential

For its continuous task of alternating electrical activity and ionic recovery, cardiac muscle membrane is well-provided with membrane current mechanisms. Some of these are pump or exchange currents which continually maintain the ionic gradients across the membrane to enable it to generate regular action potentials. These pumps and exchangers are summarized in Fig. 4.5. Others are the current mechanisms involved in the actual excitation process, some of which are controlled by activation and inactivation gates showing both

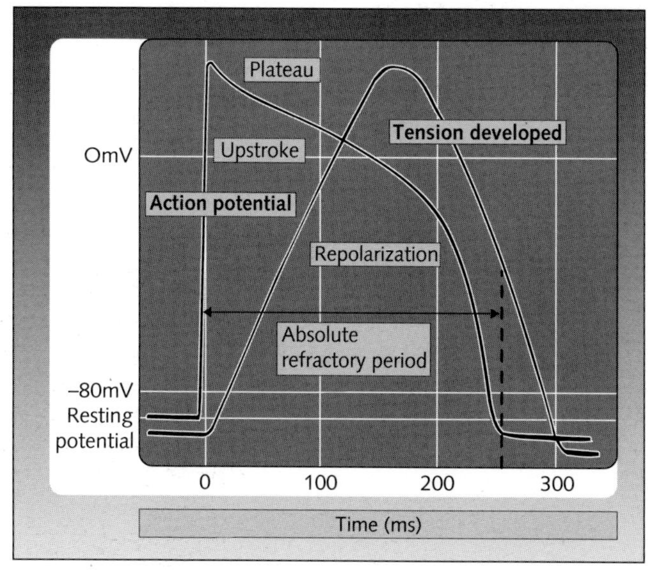

Figure 4.3
Action potential from a guinea-pig isolated ventricular cell stimulated at a rate of 2/s, showing its main phases and its time-relationship to the tension developed by the cell. The absolute refractory period associated with the long cardiac action potential is also shown.

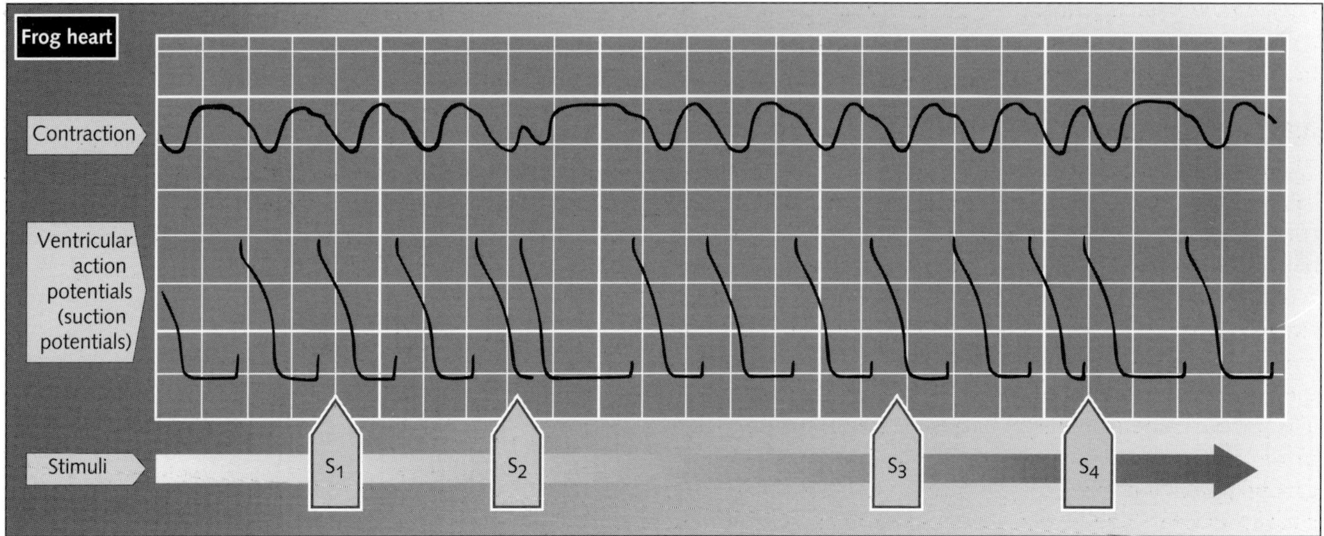

Figure 4.4
In this record of the contractions and the suction electrode potentials (equivalent to action potentials) from a spontaneously beating isolated perfused frog heart, external stimuli (arrowed) have been given to the ventricle at different points in the cycle: the first and third of these fall during the absolute refractory period and produce no further excitation but the second and fourth (S_2 and S_4) fall during the relative refractory period and excite short, extra action potentials and small extra contractions (premature beats).

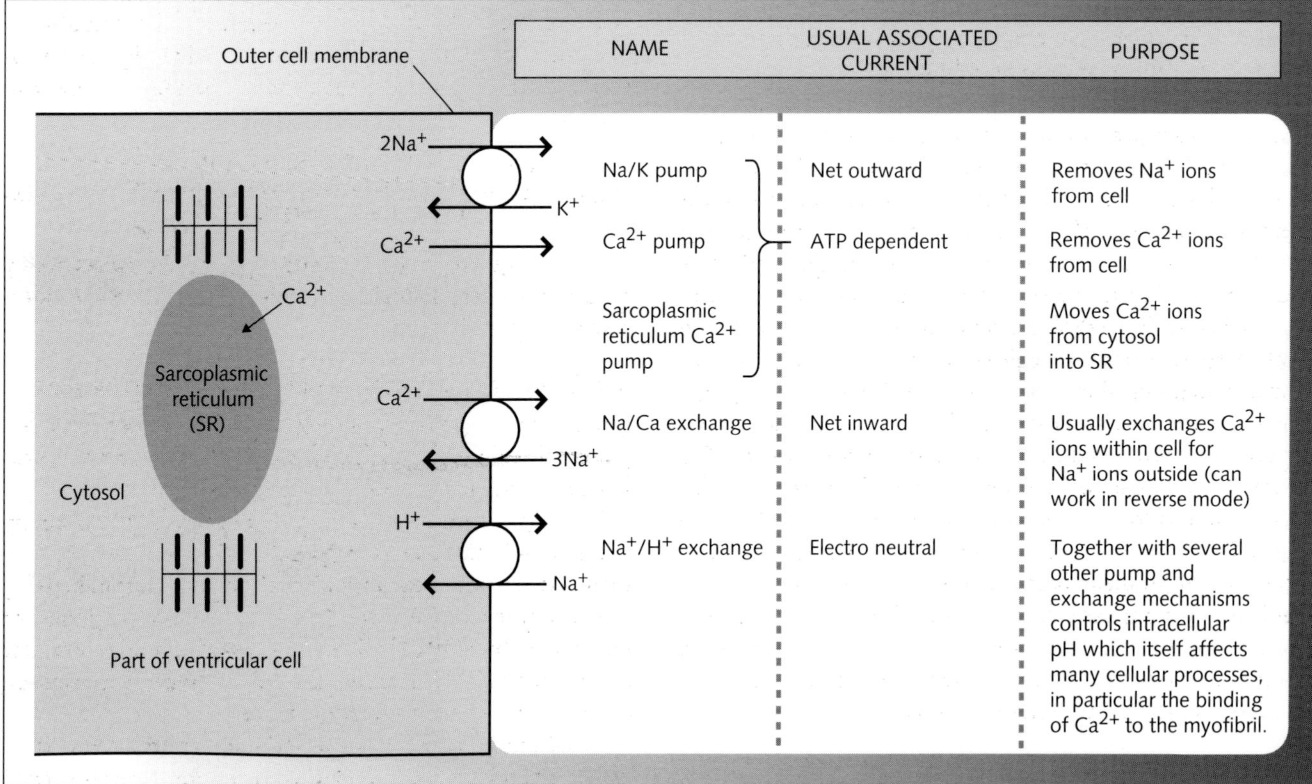

NAME	USUAL ASSOCIATED CURRENT	PURPOSE
Na/K pump	Net outward	Removes Na^+ ions from cell
Ca^{2+} pump	ATP dependent	Removes Ca^{2+} ions from cell
Sarcoplasmic reticulum Ca^{2+} pump		Moves Ca^{2+} ions from cytosol into SR
Na/Ca exchange	Net inward	Usually exchanges Ca^{2+} ions within cell for Na^+ ions outside (can work in reverse mode)
Na^+/H^+ exchange	Electro neutral	Together with several other pump and exchange mechanisms controls intracellular pH which itself affects many cellular processes, in particular the binding of Ca^{2+} to the myofibril.

Figure 4.5
The main pump and exchange mechanisms in the cardiac membrane which by their activity closely control the ionic concentrations within the cardiac cell.

time- and voltage-dependence, while others are more simply controlled and only alter with the voltage across the membrane and not with time (time-independent currents).

4.6 Resting (diastolic) potential

The development of the resting potential in the ventricular cell is essentially similar to that in other excitable cells. At rest (that is, during diastole) the membrane is much more permeable to potassium ions than to the other ions commonly found in body fluids, so, from the Nernst equation and its extension, the Goldman equation (see below) the resting membrane potential (about −80 mV in a healthy cell) is near the potassium equilibrium potential (E_K) of about −90 mV. The potassium permeability which 'sets' the resting potential in ventricular cells is the so-called inward rectifier or background potassium current, i_{K1}. The channels comprising this conductance are highly influenced by the potential across the membrane, altering their permeability to K^+ ions immediately this changes (i.e. they show voltage-dependence but no time-dependence).

4.6.1 Equilibrium potentials and the Nernst equation

The excitable nature of nerve and muscle cells, including cardiac myocytes, can be attributed to the distribution of ions on either side of the cell membrane. This imbalance results in the development of a potential difference, known as the membrane potential, between the intra- and extracellular membrane surfaces. To understand this, it is easiest to consider a simple two-compartment model separated by a membrane with pores permeable only to a single type of ion, for example, potassium. If a high concentration of a potassium salt (K^+A^-) is introduced into the left compartment and a low concentration is introduced to the right, potassium ions will start to diffuse down their concentration gradient from left to right carrying positive charge with them. The membrane is, however, impermeable to the anion (A^-) and thus a charge imbalance will develop which results in a potential difference between the two compartments (right positive to left). The greater the potential difference becomes, the harder it is for potassium ions to move against this newly generated electrical gradient. Eventually an equilibrium is reached at which the electrical gradient balances the chemical concentration gradient in the opposite direction. At this time the potassium ions are said to be in electrochemical equilibrium across the membrane. The equilibrium potential is given by equation 1, the Nernst equation for potassium ions

$$E_K = (RT/ZF)\ln\left([K^+]_{right}/[K^+]_{left}\right) \quad (1)$$

where R is the gas constant, T is the temperature (in degrees Kelvin), F is the Faraday constant and Z is the valency of the ion (one for potassium) and $[K^+]_{left}$ and $[K^+]_{right}$ represent the concentration of potassium ions in the two compartments.

The resting membrane potential

Equation 1 can be applied to biological systems. Thus, the equilibrium potential for a cell with a membrane permeable only to potassium ions is determined by the ratio of the potassium ion concentration across the membrane. The Nernst equation can be written using the notation given in equation 2:

$$E_K = (RT/ZF)\ln\left([K^+]_o/[K^+]_i\right) \quad (2)$$

where $[K^+]_i$ and $[K^+]_o$ are the concentrations of potassium ions inside and outside the cell.

If the membrane were really permeable only to K^+ ions, the resting membrane potential would be of the order of −85 mV. In practice this is rarely the case, since the cell membrane is also somewhat permeable to other biologically relevant ions such as sodium, chloride and calcium. The physiological distribution of, for example, sodium ions tends to make the inside of the cell less negative relative to the outside, thus shifting the membrane potential a little more positive than −85 mV. The resting membrane potential can be more accurately calculated from the mean of the equilibrium potentials for all the permeant ions, weighted by their relative permeabilities (P) (equation 3; modified Goldman equation)

$$E_{mem} = \frac{RT}{F}\ln\frac{P_K[K^+]_o + P_{Na}[Na^+]_o + P_{Cl}[Cl^-]_i}{P_K[K^+]_i + P_{Na}[Na^+]_i + P_{Cl}[Cl^-]_o} \quad (3)$$

In this equation P_K, P_{Na} and P_{Cl} are the permeability coefficients for potassium, sodium and chloride ions, respectively.

4.7 The upstroke of the ventricular action potential

The computer simulation in Fig. 4.6 of a ventricular action potential and the membrane currents which generate it provides guidance for the next three sections.

Once the ventricular cell membrane is depolarized by about 15 mV, that is, to about −65 mV (a process that normally occurs when excitation reaches it from neighbouring cells), a regenerative inward sodium current (i_{Na}) rapidly depolarizes it and causes the upstroke of the ventricular action potential. This current is similar to the inward sodium current of the squid giant axon and other nerve cells.

In addition to the inward sodium current, there is in cardiac muscle cells a second inward current which is carried by calcium ions (Fig. 4.6) and which has a rather more positive activation threshold (around −45 mV). It has sometimes been called the slow inward current, though it is slow only by comparison with the inward sodium current, its time to peak

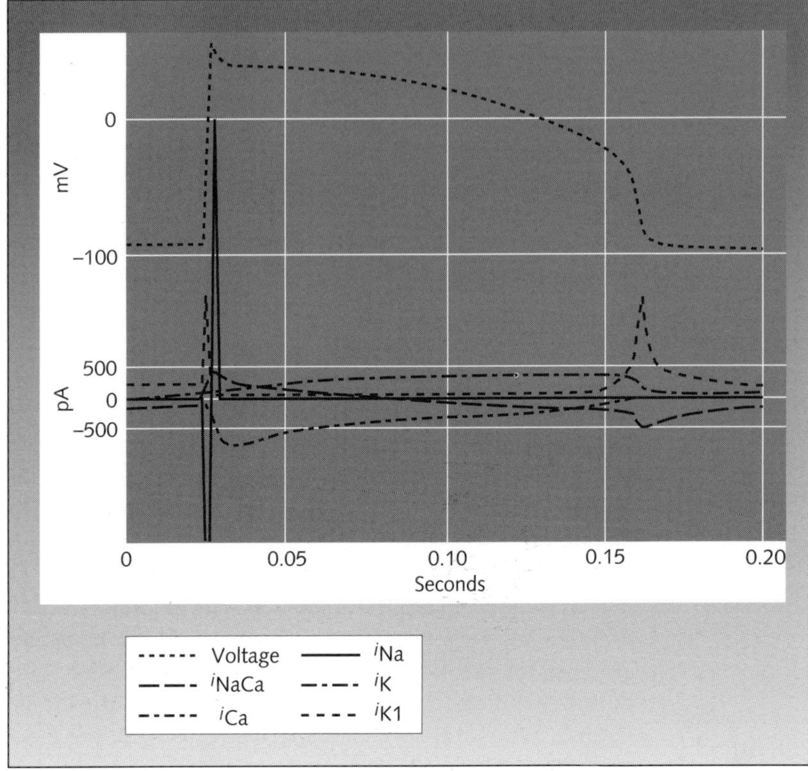

Figure 4.6
This OXSOFT HEART computer simulation shows the main membrane currents underlying the ventricular myocyte action potential. Note that the amplitude of the sodium current, i_{Na}, is so large compared to the other currents that only an eight-fold reduction of the scale would accommodate it all within the confines of this plot. Inward current plotted down screen and outward, up screen.

(a)

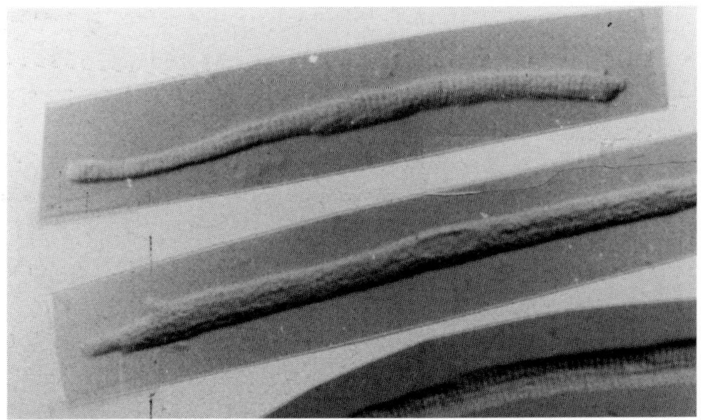

Atrium
0
mV
−80
(b)
100 ms

Figure 4.7
(a) Isolated atrial cell from a guinea-pig. Dimensions are 120 × 10 μm. (Courtesy of Dr A. Levi.) (b) Atrial action potential. Note the shorter duration and more triangular shape compared with the ventricular action potential.

in a single cardiac muscle cell being about 2 ms compared to 0.5 ms for the sodium current. This inward calcium current ($i_{Ca,L}$) makes a contribution to the upstroke, though under normal conditions in ventricular cells this is not the major one; its chief roles are as the very important trigger of further calcium release within the cell leading to the activation of contraction (Chapter 10) and as a contributor to the action potential plateau. Both i_{Na} and $i_{Ca,L}$ show voltage-dependence and also time-dependence, that is, once their voltage threshold is reached, they activate (and also inactivate) with characteristic time courses.

4.8 Plateau

In the nerve or skeletal muscle fibre, inactivation of the sodium current coupled with a slightly slower (but still rapid) increase in potassium permeability on depolarization leads to outflow of potassium ions and repolarization of the membrane within a few milliseconds, but in the ventricular cell a long depolarized plateau phase of the action potential develops after the upstroke. The sodium current is inactivated rapidly in much the same way as in the nerve fibre membrane but potassium conductance initially *decreases* markedly when the ventricular cell membrane is depolarized. The time-independent or background potassium current (i_{K1}) which during diastole maintains the membrane potential near E_K becomes much smaller when the membrane is depolarized, so that at the level of the plateau (around 0 mV), there is little outward (repolarizing) current from this source. What there is, is counterbalanced by three small amounts of inward currents:

- A small but important inward sodium (i_{Na}) 'window' current flows caused by the slight overlap of the m (activation) and h (inactivation) curves at these potentials, giving an inward current through sodium channels which have not been inactivated.
- The calcium current ($i_{Ca,L}$) also plays a part in maintaining the plateau: it takes about 100 ms to inactivate at 0 mV, so it contributes inward current to the maintenance of the first half of the plateau.
- Overlapping the inward calcium current and continuing after it has inactivated is a further inward current associated with the extrusion from the cardiac cell of the Ca^{2+} ions that have entered. Such exchange is one of the important continuous maintenance strategies of cardiac cell membranes (see Fig. 4.5); the calcium ions are extruded in exchange for sodium ions, and since three Na^{+} ions enter the cell for each Ca^{2+} ion which leaves, this exchange process gives a net inward sodium/calcium exchange current (i_{NaCa}) which contributes to the maintenance of the plateau.

This mechanism of maintaining the plateau by reducing outward (repolarizing) current and balancing it by small but important inward (depolarizing) currents uses very small amounts of current flow. It is a much more energy-efficient solution than the possible alternative one of countering a large outward potassium conductance by an equally large inward current (e.g. by delaying the inactivation of the sodium current).

4.9 Repolarization

In the ventricular cells of many, but not all, mammalian species an outward time-dependent potassium current is switched on by depolarization as it is in nerve fibres, but its activation is very much slower. After some 250 ms, the inward currents have declined and this outward current (i_K), if present, speeds up repolarization of the membrane. The background potassium current, i_{K1}, will in any case contribute progressively more to repolarization as it proceeds and this current becomes larger again at more negative potentials.

4.10 The importance of i_{K1}

It is interesting to consider why the ventricular cell has developed the complexity of an i_{K1} system which has to be switched off during each action potential. Its importance is in setting and maintaining the diastolic resting potential. It stabilizes the cell membrane against random excitation which can arise ectopically and lead to arrhythmias (see Chapter 7). A sizeable potassium conductance acts against stray depolarizations before these can depolarize the membrane as far as the threshold of i_{Na}. It is significant that in pacemaking cells of the SA node, where membrane stability is *not* required, i_{K1} is absent (see Chapter 5).

4.11 Electrical activity of the atrium

Atrial fibres are slimmer than ventricular ones but of comparable length (Fig. 4.7a). Atrial action potentials are of much shorter duration than those of ventricular cells (80 ms compared with 250 ms) with hardly any plateau (Fig. 4.7b). An additional time-dependent potassium current which is not found in ventricle cells is responsible for the initial phase of repolarization in the atrial cells of many mammalian species. This is the transient outward current (i_{to}) which is activated with a rapid time-course by depolarizations to potentials positive to −30 mV. It thus provides a significant amount of repolarizing current right from the start of the action potential. There is also relatively more potassium current at depolarized potentials in atrial cells than in ventricular ones and these two factors account for the short, triangular form of the atrial action potential.

5 Cardiac cellular electrophysiology: pacemaking and conducting tissue

5.1 The sinoatrial node

As was shown in Fig. 3.4, the sinoatrial (SA) node is located in the wall of the right atrium near the points of entry of the superior and inferior venae cavae. In Fig. 5.1, the right atrium of a rabbit has been spread out in a dissecting dish with the superior vena cava opened up to show the SA node.

A considerable amount is known about the organization of the SA node itself from recordings taken from cells in the intact node or in smaller preparations of nodal tissue with a single microelectrode. There is a central region which is normally the first to fire at each heart beat (Fig. 5.2).

Undamaged isolated SA node cells from a rabbit heart (and those of other species which have been isolated) are spindle-shaped, about 10 µm wide and 50–150 µm long with a central nucleus (Fig. 5.3a). Each cell will beat spontaneously when superfused with Tyrode solution at 37°C. Recordings can be taken from such cells using the patch-clamp technique in the whole cell mode (see Fig. 4.1). The cell will continue to beat vigorously, pivoting round the patch-clamp electrode sealed to its membrane. A typical record of the spontaneous firing of such a cell is shown in Fig. 5.3b. There are several differences between this electrical activity and that of a ventricular cell:

1 The spontaneous pacemaker depolarization extending from the maximum diastolic potential of –65 to –45 mV, the beginning of the action potential upstroke.

2 The less negative maximum diastolic potential, –65 mV compared with –85 mV ventricular cell resting potential.

3 The action potential upstroke rises more slowly: it is essentially a calcium upstroke, supported by the inward calcium current $i_{Ca,L}$. In some SA node cells there is a contribution from inward sodium current, i_{Na}, but this is not essential for firing which continues with little alteration if the sodium current is blocked (Fig. 5.3c).

4 The action potential has no plateau.

5.2 Pacemaking in sinoatrial node cells

5.2.1 Maximum diastolic potential of the sinoatrial node cell

SA node cells lack the stabilizing background potassium conductance, i_{K1}, found in ventricular cells and they are also very small cells. Thus the passage of a very small amount of current, just a few picoamps (1 pA = 10^{-12} A) will alter their membrane potential. Their maximum diastolic potential of about –65 mV implies a relatively high background Na^+ permeability relative to K^+ permeability.

Three membrane current mechanisms contribute to the SA nodal pacemaker depolarization:

5.2.2 The hyperpolarization-activated inward current, i_f

This membrane current has unusual ('funny') but very appropriate properties for maintaining pacemaker activity: the more the membrane is hyperpolarized, the more of this inward (and therefore depolarizing) current is activated. At positive potentials, such as those reached during the action potential, i_f is rapidly deactivated, but the deactivation is removed as the membrane repolarizes again to the maximum diastolic potential. Thus all is ready for i_f to be activated again during the next pacemaker depolarization.

Figure 5.4a gives voltage clamp records from an isolated SA node cell which show how the activation of i_f increases with increasing levels of hyperpolarization and how it switches off very rapidly at +20 mV.

The usual pacemaker range of SA node cells (–65 to –45 mV) only overlaps the very bottom of the i_f activation curve which extends to very much more negative potentials. This, coupled with the very slow activation rate of i_f, means that often rather little i_f is activated during the SA nodal pacemaker depolarization. Moreover, when i_f is blocked (by 2 mmol/l caesium or other blockers), SA node cells can and do continue to beat, although at a slower rate than before the blocker was applied (Fig. 5.4b).

i_f can be considered as an important contributor to the more negative part of the SA node pacemaker depolarization and as a safety factor ready in reserve to depolarize the membrane ever more strongly, the more negative the maximum diastolic potential becomes. It is thought to be important in maintaining the beating of the cells at the periphery of the node which are inevitably subjected to the passive flow of hyperpolarizing current from the atrial cells to which they are connected and which have more negative diastolic potentials of about –80 mV (see Fig. 4.7b).

5.2.3 Calcium currents

An important contribution to the later part of the SA node pacemaker depolarization comes from inward calcium current, the long-lasting calcium current, $i_{Ca,L}$, which con-

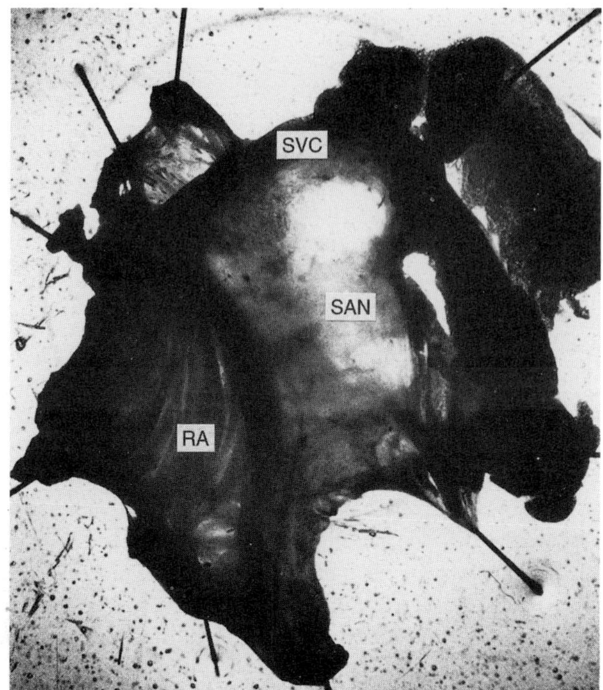

Figure 5.1
The right atrial region of a rabbit heart was cut open along the venae cavae. The opened right atrium was pinned out to the left so that the sinoatrial node can be seen (the transparent area). The rabbit SA node measures about 10 × 4 mm. SVC, superior vena cava; RA, right atrium; SAN, sinoatrial node.

tributes to depolarization at potentials positive to −55 mV. This current is shown in the voltage clamp records in Fig. 5.5. Increase in this calcium current contributes to the great increases in rate brought about by catecholamines (see Chapter 12).

Another calcium current, the transient calcium current, $i_{Ca,T}$ probably contributes some inward depolarizing current to the pacemaker potential. Its threshold of inactivation is more negative (about −55 mV) than that of $i_{Ca,L}$, so it may be involved in more of the pacemaker potential. As its name implies, it is, however, rapidly inactivated and the extent of its participation in pacemaking is not yet fully determined. It is not increased by catecholamines.

5.2.4 Inward background current and the decay of time-dependent potassium current

The pacemaker depolarization continues in SA node cells when i_f is blocked. It is then controlled by the decay of the time-dependent potassium current i_K. In Fig. 5.5 the decrease of this potassium current when the potential is returned to −40 mV after positive voltage clamp pulses can be seen as decaying current 'tails' whose time-course is comparable to that of a pacemaker depolarization. Decay of an outward current cannot, however, bring about depolarization by itself; it must be set against some kind of inward current (see note on Goldman equation in Chapter 4). This mode of pacemaking can be seen in depolarized Purkinje fibres (see Fig. 5.8c) or atrial cells depolarized by an applied inward current. The nature of the inward background current or 'leak' current in SA node cells is not yet certain, since such currents are difficult to record in isolation. It is very probably a 'leak' current carried by Na^+ ions ($i_{b,Na}$, inward background current).

The mechanisms of SA nodal pacing are summarized in Fig. 5.6.

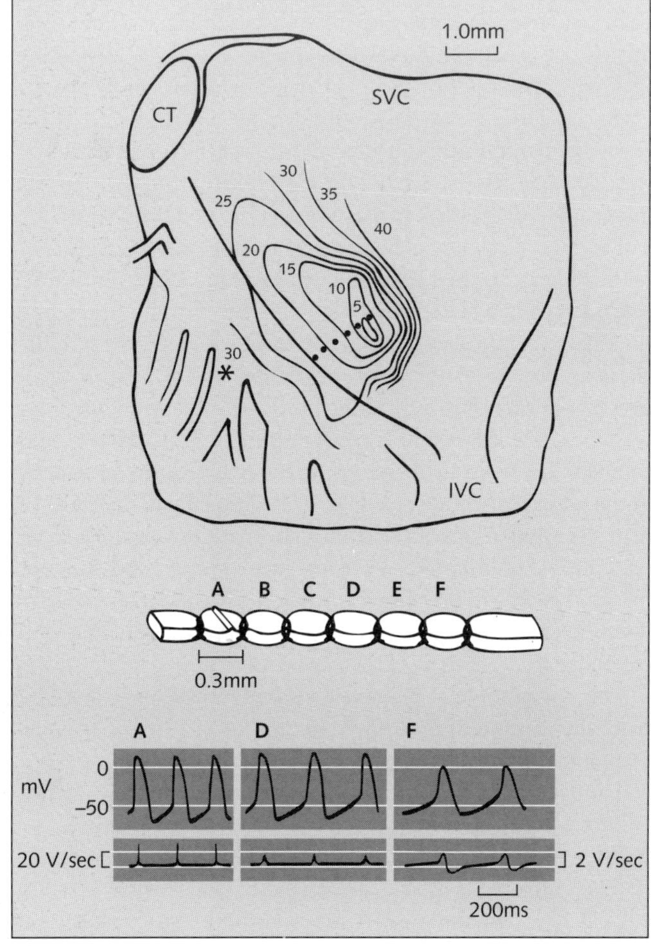

Figure 5.2
Map of the activation pattern in a whole sinus node preparation: action potentials in a total of 53 cells in a sinoatrial node were recorded consecutively by microelectrode impalements. The activation times were calculated relative to that of an atrial cell impaled by another electrode (star) and plotted as isochronal lines at 5 ms intervals. The location of a strip of tissue then cut from the node is shown by the line of black dots; each dot represents a length of this strip which was then separated by ligatures to give the small preparations A–F. Spontaneous activity recorded from A, D and F is also shown. (From Kodama, I. & Boyett, M.R. (1985). *Pflügers Archiv* **404**, 214–226, with permission.) CT, crista terminalis; SVC, IVC, superior and inferior venae cavae.

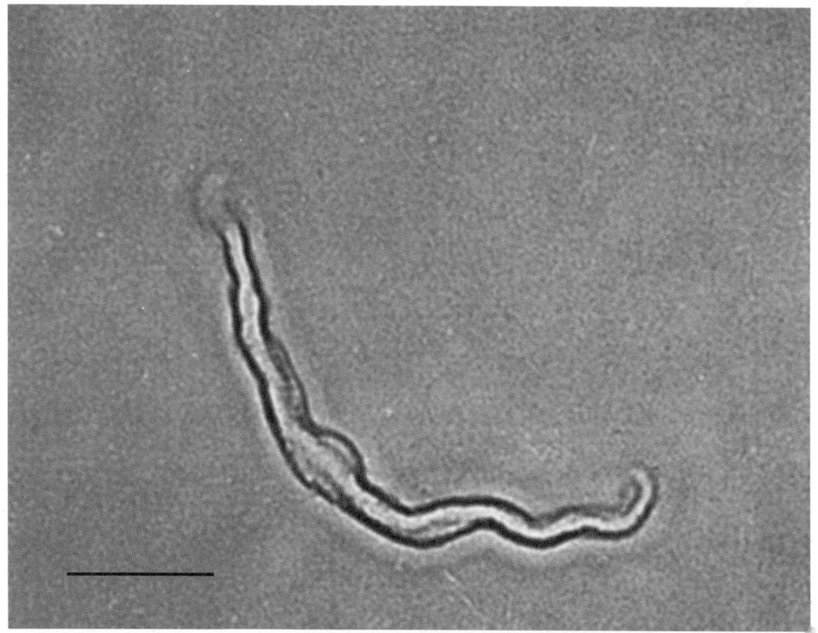

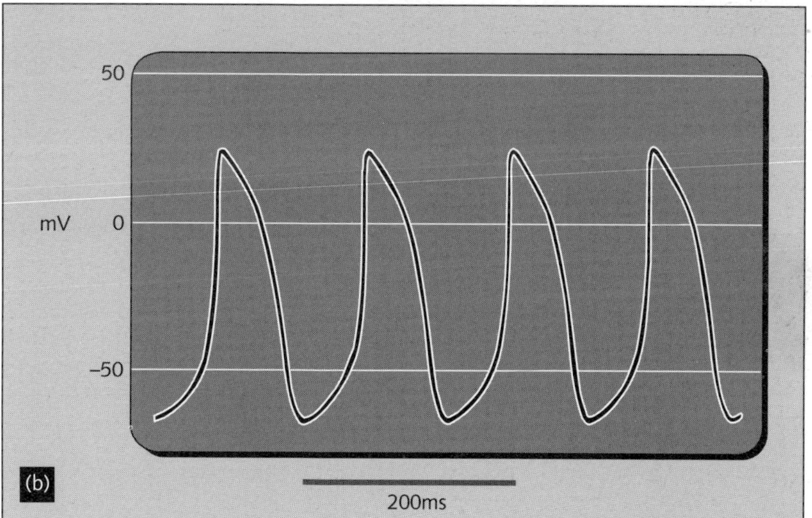

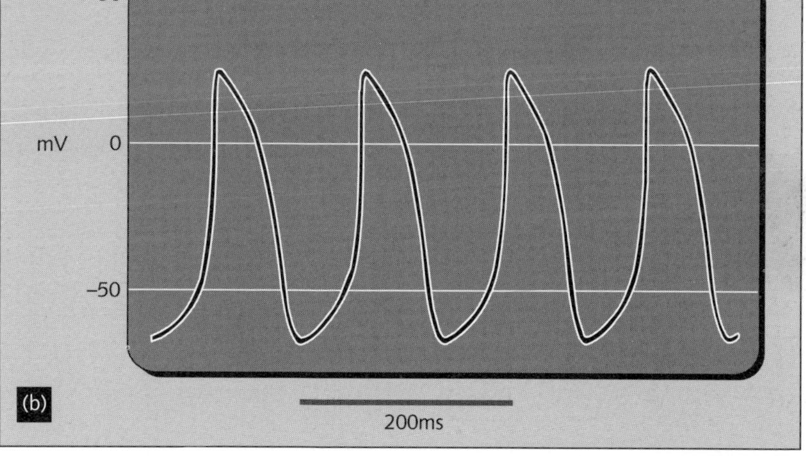

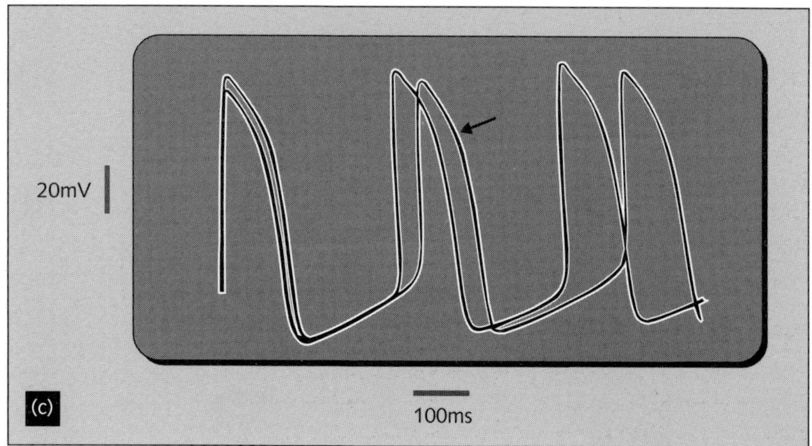

Figure 5.3
(a) Isolated sinoatrial node cell of rabbit. The cells are spindle-shaped with a prominent central nucleus. Length bar 25 μm. (b) Spontaneous electrical activity of a single sinoatrial node cell. From the maximum diastolic potential of about –65 mV, the pacemaker potential depolarizes the membrane to the beginning of the action potential upstroke at about –45 mV. (c) Effect of tetrodotoxin (arrowed trace) which abolishes the inward sodium current component which contributes to the activity of most sinoatrial node cells: the upstroke velocity is reduced but the remaining inward current (calcium) can support the action potential upstroke and firing continues at a slightly slower rate.

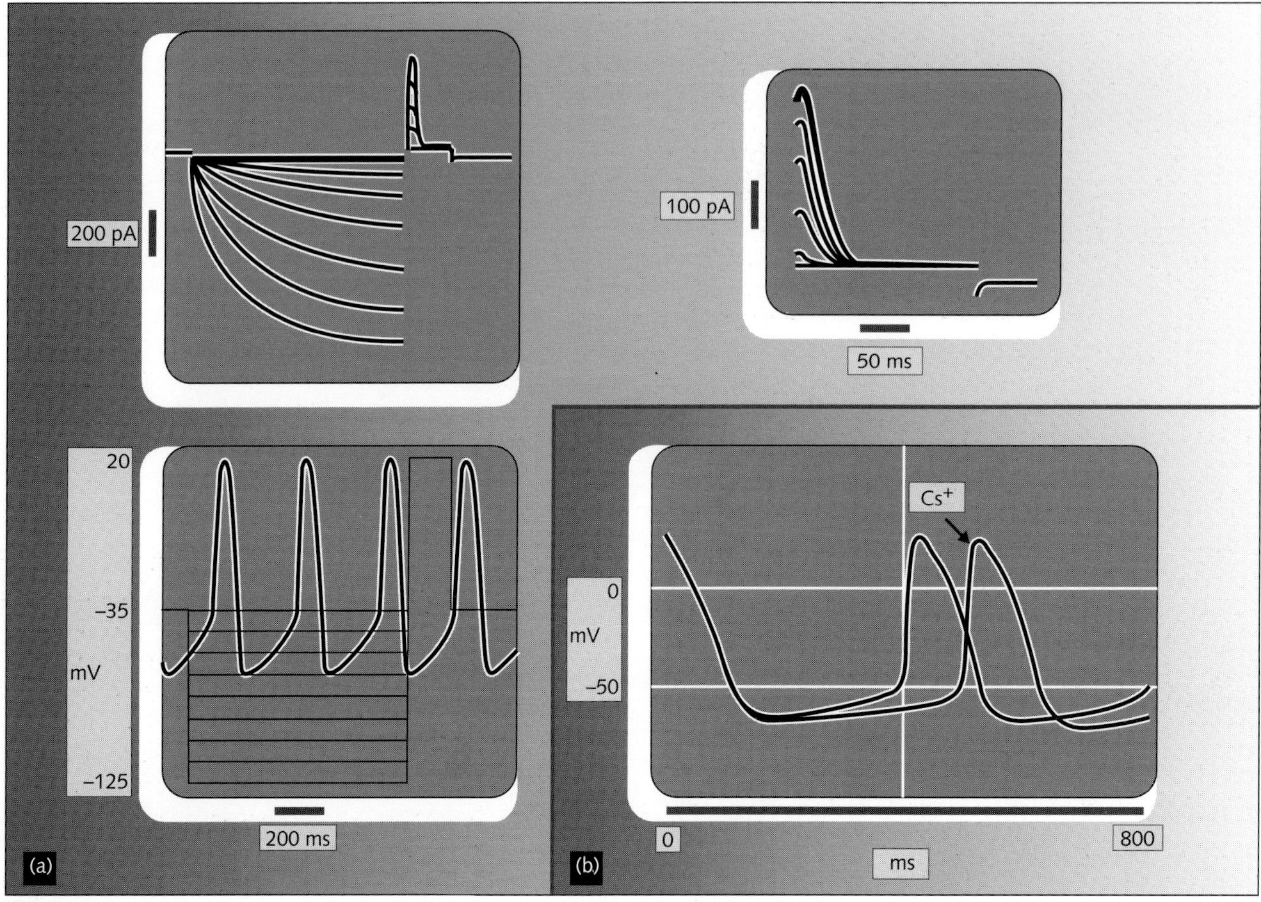

Figure 5.4
(a) For these voltage clamp recordings, the membrane potential of a sinoatrial node cell was held at −35 mV and the cell then given 1s hyperpolarizing pulses to progressively more negative potentials followed by a 100 ms positive clamp pulse to +20 mV in each case before being returned to −35 mV. All the voltage pulses have been superimposed (bottom record in (a)), as has also the (unclamped) spontaneous activity of the cell to show the level of the clamp pulses relative to the pacemaker and action potentials. The membrane currents recorded during each clamp pulse are shown above the voltage traces; they have also been superimposed on one another. The downward deflections of the current traces during each hyperpolarizing clamp pulse show activation of the hyperpolarization-activated inward current (i_f); the further the membrane is hyperpolarized, the more of this current develops. After each hyperpolarizing clamp pulse, a voltage pulse to +20 mV was given. The rapid switch-off of i_f is seen as quickly decaying 'tails' of current (enlarged top right). (b) In 2 mmol/l caesium chloride (which blocks the hyperpolarization-activated inward current, i_f) the spontaneous firing of a sinoatrial node cell is slowed but not stopped.

5.3 Conduction pathways through the atrium

Although special conduction pathways through the atrium for the excitation wave have been described, there is no conclusive evidence for them and it is probable that excitation travels across the atrium along ordinary atrial fibres at a rate of about 1 m/s.

5.4 The atrioventricular node

The atrioventricular (AV) node was first identified in 1906 by the Japanese histologist Tawara. It is approximately 22 mm long, 10 mm wide and 3 mm thick in the human and divided into three discrete zones (Fig. 5.7a). It forms the only conducting pathway between the atrial muscle and the bundle of His and hence the ventricles, except in abnormal circumstances when an extra connection exists which can provoke arrhythmias and must be removed (Chapter 9).

It is in the AV node that the considerable delay to the excitation wave (100 ms) occurs; this allows time for blood to move from atria to ventricles (Chapter 3). The excitation front is slowed from 0.5 m/s in atrial muscle to 0.05 m/s within the AV node. When impulses are extinguished within

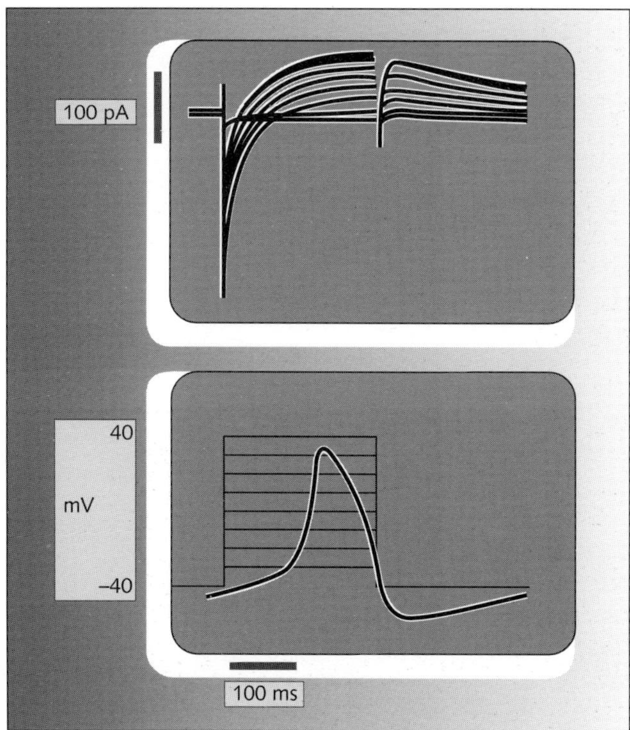

Figure 5.5
Voltage clamp depolarizations from a holding potential of –40 mV up to +40 mV (once again superimposed together with unclamped electrical activity from the same cell) rapidly activate inward calcium current, the downward deflections in the current records. This inactivates within the first 100 ms of the clamp pulse and the activation of outward potassium current, i_K (upward deflections) is then evident. When the membrane potential is returned to 0 mV after each pulse, the potassium current decays away as a slow 'tail', the time-course of which is comparable to that of the pacemaker depolarization.

the AV node and so fail to excite the ventricles, the condition is known as heart block (Chapter 7), and it may be complete or partial.

AV node cells are smaller than ventricular cells (Fig. 5.7b). Their electrical properties show similarities to those of SA node cells. The action potential upstroke has a low upstroke velocity and is little affected by tetrodotoxin—characteristics indicating that, as in SA node, inward calcium current is the main current underlying it. The relatively slow upstroke and smaller cell size account for the low conduction velocity of excitation within the AV node.

AV node cells have well-developed latent powers of rhythmicity and can take over impulse initiation if impulses from the SA node fail to reach them.

5.5 The Purkinje fibres

5.5.1 Location and arrangement

The Purkinje fibres form the right and left branches of the bundle of His, leading from the AV node down the ventricular septum and turning back along the inner surface of the ventricles as the ramifying Purkinje network (Fig. 3.4). To ensure almost synchronous excitation of the ventricles, conduction within the Purkinje fibres is fast (5 m/s; Chapter 3). To this end the Purkinje fibres are arranged in cylinders (Fig. 5.8a). In some species (sheep and cattle) the Purkinje cells are very large and empty-looking but in humans the Purkinje cells differ little in appearance from normal ventricular cells.

The action potential of the Purkinje fibre is similar to that of the ventricular cell, though the plateau is at a rather more negative potential (Fig. 5.8b) and the duration of the action potentials is rather longer, giving protection against possible re-excitation from the ventricle.

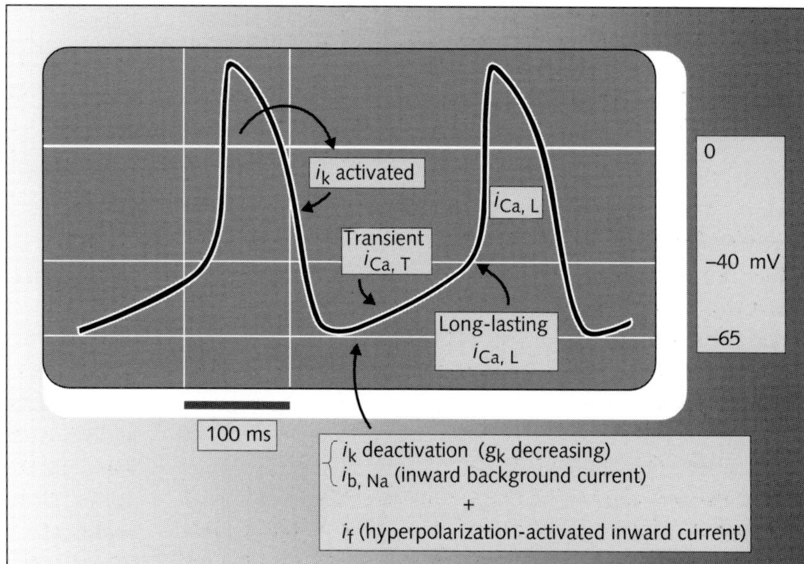

Figure 5.6
Summary of the sinoatrial pacemaker mechanism. i_K: outward potassium current; $i_{Ca,L}$, $i_{Ca,T}$: long-lasting and transient inward calcium currents; i_f: hyperpolarization activated inward current; $i_{b,Na}$: inward background current. This scheme does not include other background (time-independent) currents which may influence pacemaking (e.g. currents resulting from Na^+/K^+ pump activity (outward) or Na^+/Ca^{2+} exchange (inward) nor the sustained inward current present in some cells which seems to be carried by Na^+ ions through $i_{Ca,L}$ channels.

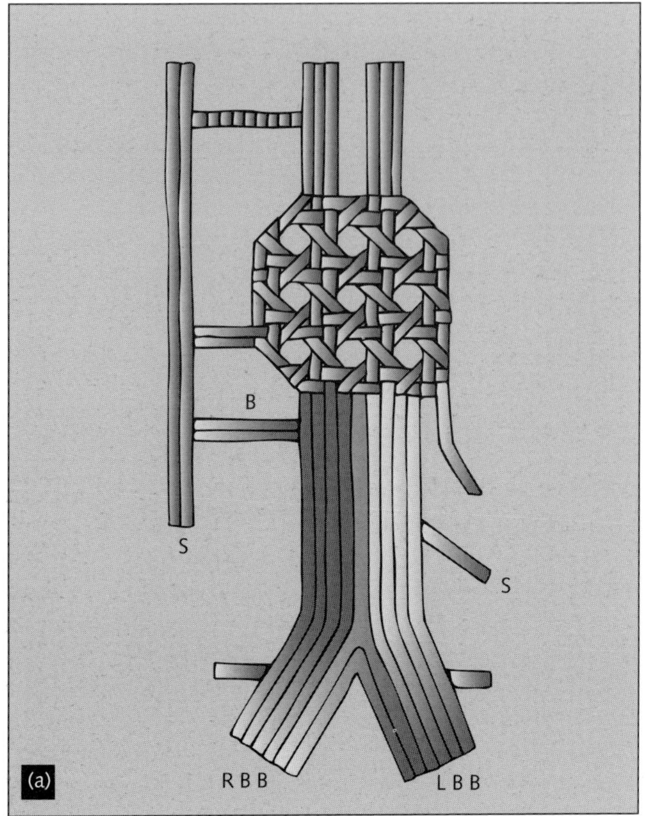

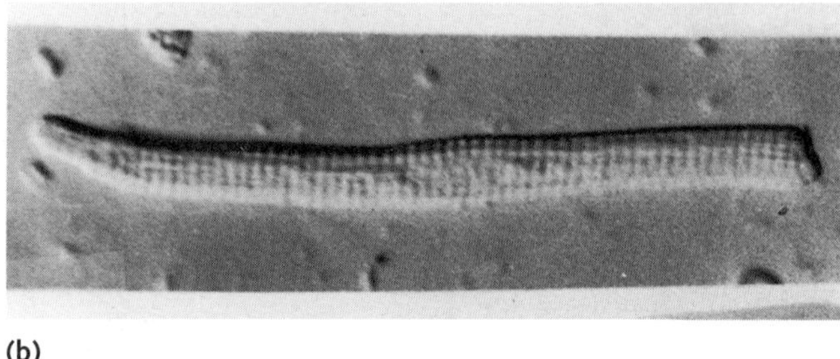

(b)

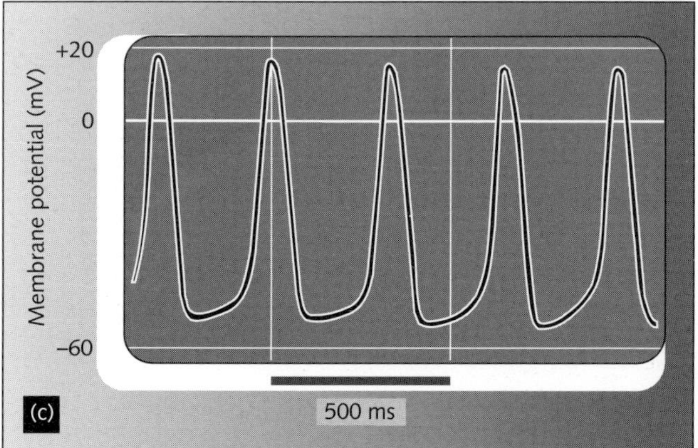

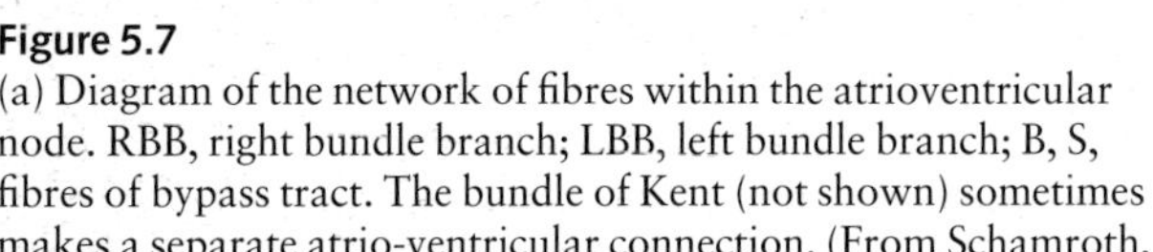

Figure 5.7
(a) Diagram of the network of fibres within the atrioventricular node. RBB, right bundle branch; LBB, left bundle branch; B, S, fibres of bypass tract. The bundle of Kent (not shown) sometimes makes a separate atrio-ventricular connection. (From Schamroth, L. (1971) *The Disorders of Cardiac Rhythm*. Blackwell Scientific Publications, Oxford.) (b) An isolated atrioventricular node cell (cell dimensions c. 100 × 10 μm). (c) Electrical activity of an AV nodal cell. ((b) and (c) Courtesy of Dr A. Levi.)

5.5.2 Pacemaking in Purkinje fibres

Purkinje fibres can show pacemaker activity at a rate of about 40/min (Fig. 5.8b). In the whole heart, such pacemaker activity will only manifest itself under conditions of heart block, for normally the Purkinje fibres will be excited at a much higher rate by impulses arriving through the AV node. The pacemaker depolarization of the Purkinje fibre extends over the potential range −90 to −60 mV, much more negative than that of the SA node cell. The membrane current underlying it is the hyperpolarization-activated inward current, i_f, which has already been described in connection with SA nodal pacing. The Purkinje fibre pacemaker depolarization from −90 to −60 mV lies in the middle of the i_f activation range and its slower rate than that of SA nodal pacing corresponds to the slow rate of activation of i_f.

The other two contributors to SA nodal pacemaking, inward calcium current and the time-dependent decay of potassium current, normally play no role in Purkinje fibre pacemaking: −60 mV is still considerably negative to calcium current thresholds and i_K decays very rapidly at negative potentials, too fast to control this slow rate of pacemaking. In depolarized Purkinje fibres, however, a mode of pacemaking can be observed controlled by the decay of i_K set against inward depolarizing current (Fig. 5.8c), as occurs in SA node cells.

5.6 Artificial pacemakers

The first permanent artificial pacemaker was implanted in 1959 and there has since been rapid development of this form of treatment so that present-day pacemakers are quickly inserted and are small and long-lasting. They are provided when there is serious risk of bradycardia because of heart block or SA node disease. They are usually implanted via the veins and the electrodes positioned to make contact with the endocardium at the base of the right ventricle, where they stimulate the heart muscle with short-duration (0.5 ms) pulses, programmed either at a fixed rate or, in the more sophisticated models, given only when the heart rate falls below a certain value.

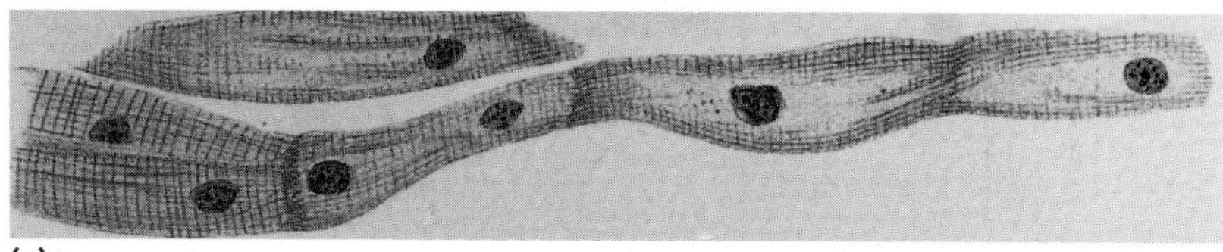

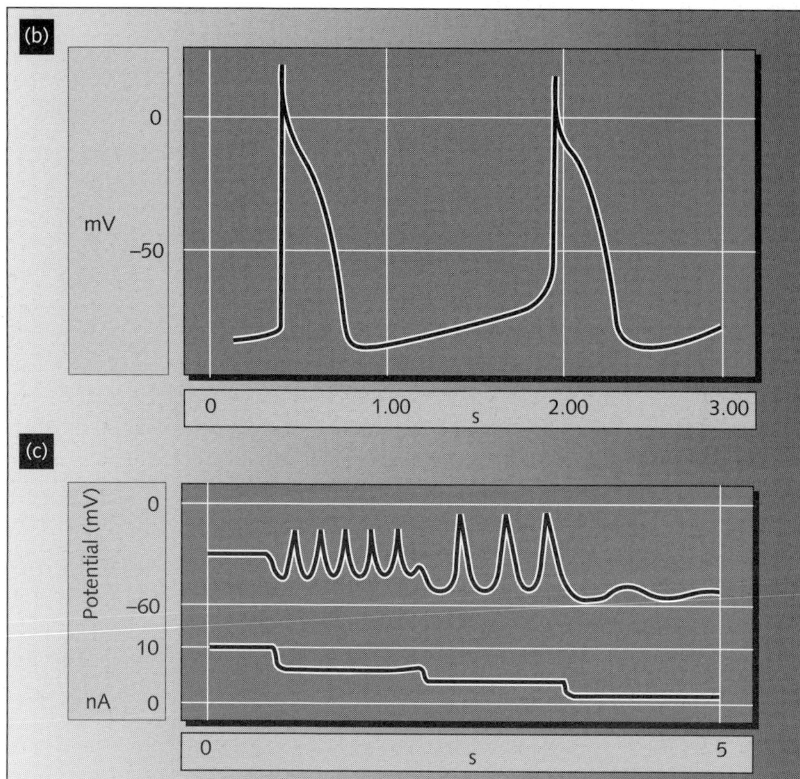

Figure 5.8
(a) Drawing of part of a Purkinje fibre from a dog heart; each cell is c. 75 × 20 μm. (From Tawara, S. (1906) *Das Reizleitungssystem des Säugetierherzens*. Gustav Fischer, Jena.) (b) Electrical activity in a pacemaking Purkinje fibre cell. (c) Pacemaker activity in depolarized Purkinje fibres. *Lower trace*: current applied to hyperpolarize this depolarized fibre. (From Noble, D. (1979) *The Initiation of the Heartbeat*, 2nd edn. Oxford University Press, Oxford, with permission.)

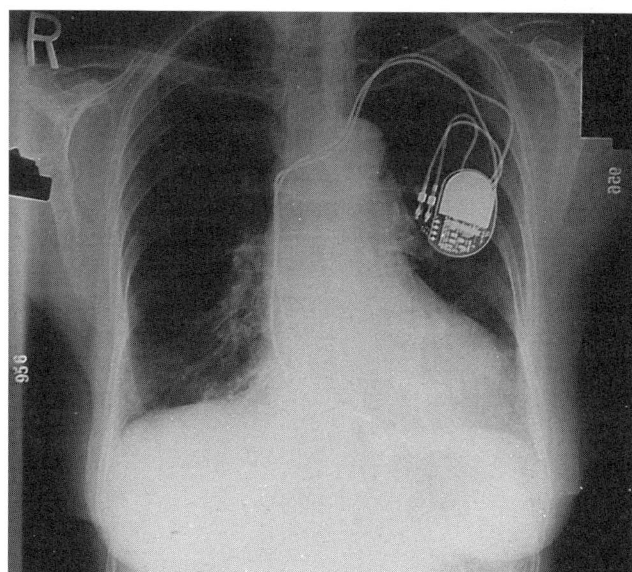

Figure 5.9
Chest X-ray showing a dual chamber rate-response pacemaker (implanted for carotid sinus hypersensitivity) in place. Under local anaesthetic, the leads are inserted via the left subclavian vein to the right ventricle and the right atrium. They are connected to the battery powered generator which is implanted in a left pre-pectoral pocket. (Courtesy of Dr C.J. Plummer, Freeman Hospital, Newcastle upon Tyne.)

Recent developments include the dual-chamber pacemaker (Fig. 5.9), which can sense and synchronize atrial and ventricular activity, and generators capable of delivering high-energy shocks for defibrillation when needed. Whereas at first the batteries in implanted pacemakers had to be replaced every 6 months, they now last between 5 and 15 years (see also Chapter 9).

6 The electrocardiogram

6.1 General features of the electrocardiogram

In the 100 years since A.D. Waller first demonstrated that the electrical changes during each heart beat could be detected at the surface of the body, electrocardiography has grown into a large and clinically very important subject. Real understanding of the electrocardiogram (ECG) depends on being able to relate the wave patterns recorded externally to what is happening at the cellular level.

The membrane currents underlying the electrical impulse of cardiac muscle cells have been described in Chapters 4 and 5. The flow of current ahead of the impulse, which depolarizes the next region of membrane so that it, in its turn, reaches the threshold for action potential firing, was shown diagrammatically in Fig. 3.1. The spread of excitation is essentially the same in cardiac muscle as in nerve, since the inside of each myocyte is electrically connected to that of others by the low-resistance nexi within the gap junctions (Fig. 3.2).

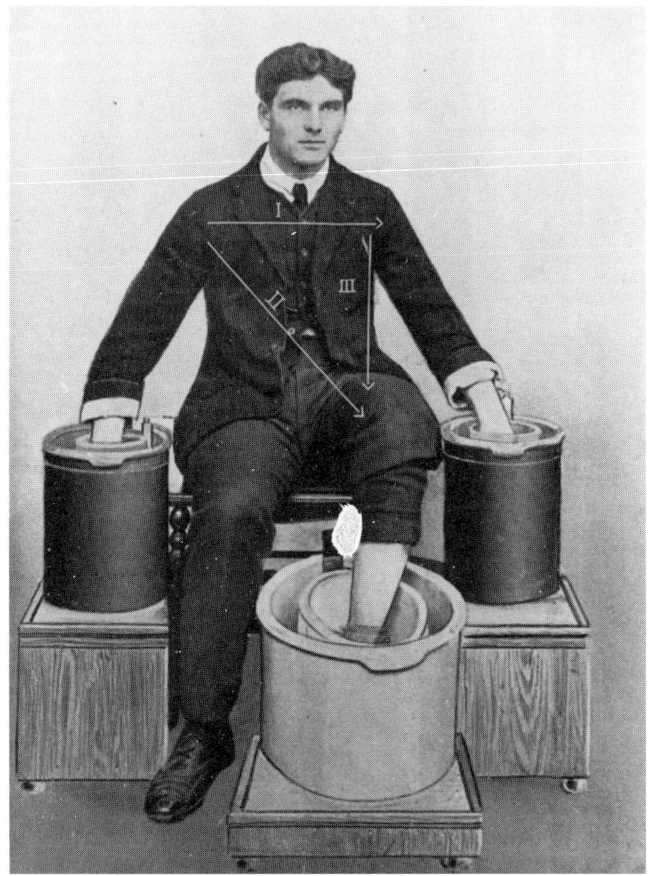

Figure 6.1
Early method of recording the electrocardiogram. (Lewis, T. (1925) *Mechanism and Graphic Registration of the Heartbeat*. Shaw & Sons, London.)

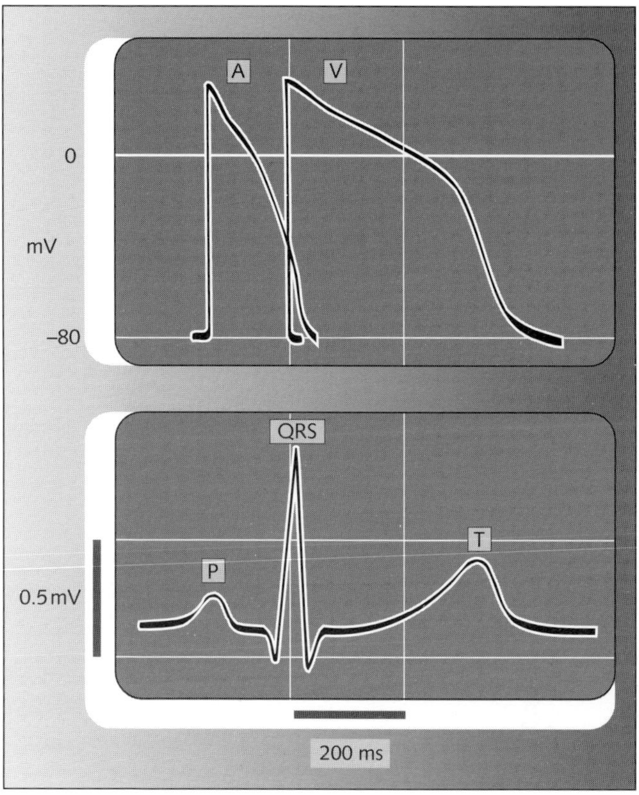

Figure 6.2
Relationship of the action potentials from an individual atrial and an individual ventricular cell (above) to electrocardiogram (below).

A recording electrode outside an excitable membrane can pick up voltage changes associated with the current which flows outside the cell during the passage of an action potential. Such changes can even be picked up at some distance from the firing nerve or muscle, particularly when, as is the case for heart excitation, many fibres are firing almost synchronously and the intervening space is occupied by the con-

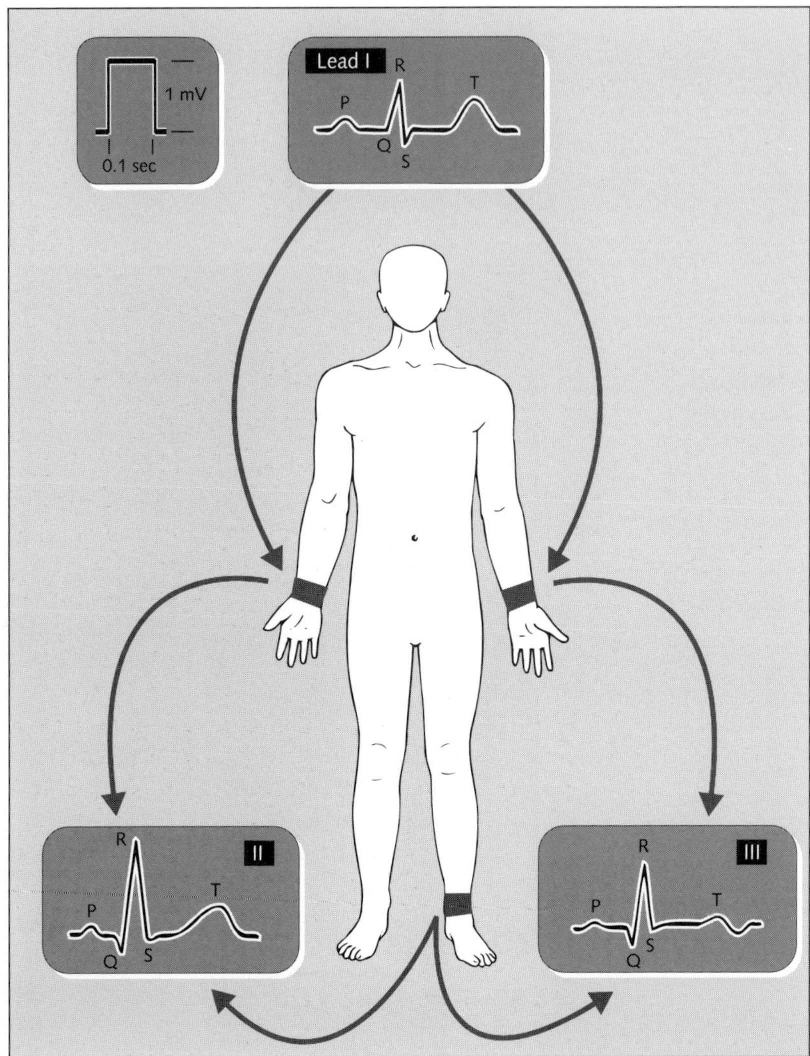

Figure 6.3
The standard limb leads for electrocardiogram recording and the normal records obtained from them.

ducting salt solutions of the body tissues. Early recording of the electrocardiogram or ECG involved cumbersome equipment (Fig. 6.1) but the records obtained were much the same as those from modern miniaturized recorders using smaller electrode plates applied to the skin with high-conductance electrode jelly.

The fastest and most prominent deflection of an ECG (Fig. 6.2) is the triphasic QRS complex, which is the extracellular record of the upstrokes of the ventricular action potentials as depolarization occurs in each cell of the ventricle in quick succession. The repolarization phase of the ventricular action potentials appears in the ECG about 200–300 ms later as the much slower and smaller T wave.

The relationship of the ECG deflections to the action potentials in the cardiac muscle itself depends partly on the size of the muscle mass firing so that the signals from the smaller amount of atrial muscle appear smaller than do those from the larger mass of ventricular muscle. Thus atrial depolarization appears in the body-surface ECG as the P wave, which is a much smaller deflection than the QRS, and sinoatrial (SA) and atrioventricular (AV) nodal activity give no visible deflection in the ECG trace. Repolarization of the atria (which might be expected to give a smaller version of the T wave) is masked in the mammalian ECG by the simultaneous QRS complex.

The relationship of the ECG to an individual atrial and

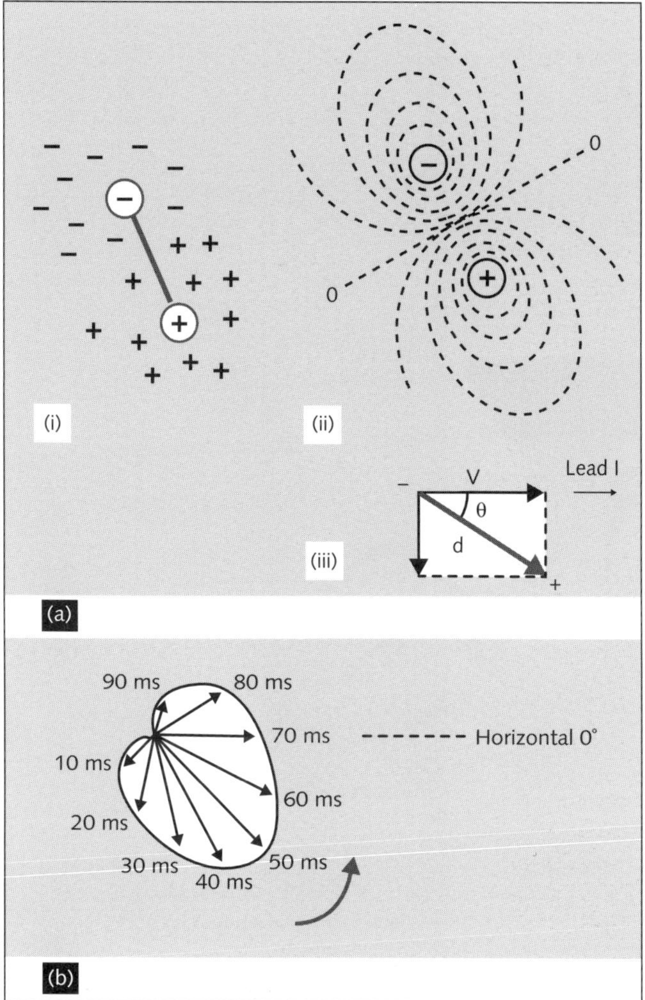

Figure 6.4
(a) Illustration of an electrical dipole and of how an electrical vector is derived. (i) Representation of two diffuse groups of opposite charges by a dipole; (ii) equipotential lines around an electrical dipole. Zero potential runs across the middle of the dipole, current flows at right angles to this; (iii) resolution of a cardiac dipole vector (thick arrow d) into two components at right angles (thin arrows). The length of arrow d is proportional to vector magnitude. The voltage difference (V) detected by Lead I depends on angle θ since $V = d \times \text{cosine}\ \theta$. (b) Changes in size and direction of the cardiac dipole vector in the frontal plane as depolarization spreads through the ventricles. (Redrawn from Levick, J.R. (1995) *An Introduction to Cardiovascular Physiology*, 2nd edn. Butterworth Heinemann, with permission.)

ventricular action potential is shown in Fig. 6.2. Notice that the ECG is a very much smaller signal than are transmembrane action potentials, about 0.5 mV compared to about 100 mV, and that waves are only recorded when the potential is changing across the cardiac muscle membranes. Thus the normal ECG trace is flat during diastole and also during the plateau phase of the action potential, i.e. between the QRS and T waves. If this is not the case, it is a sign that something is wrong (see section 6.3.1 below).

6.2 Recording the ECG

ECGs can be recorded from the standard limb leads of Einthoven on both arms and the left leg. Since the heart is oriented with its apex pointing towards the left leg, these points form a triangle round it, known as Einthoven's triangle. (Einthoven was a Dutch physicist who invented a sensitive amplifier, the string galvanometer, which, at the beginning of this century, gave the first good records of the ECG.)

Though all recording configurations show the general pattern of ECG deflections already described, there are certain consistent differences between them which are shown in Fig. 6.3 and summarized below:

I between the two arms: all the waves are positive but are smaller than with the following configuration.

II between right arm and left leg: this has the largest P, R and S waves, with small downward Q and S waves.

III between left arm and left leg: this configuration does not detect the P wave well and the T wave is also very small.

ECGs are also recorded from leads placed round the chest wall (usually six in number).

6.3 What the ECG can reveal

Study of ECG patterns from the various standard lead positions in health and disease allows accurate and detailed detection of abnormalities of cardiac excitation. These may arise from damage to the working myocardium or from aberrant behaviour of the conducting tissue; sometimes both occur together.

6.3.1 Detection of damage to the heart muscle

The electrical situation when the ECG is being recorded at the body surface is quite complex. During excitation, the heart can be considered as a dipole, that is, an electrical system oppositely charged in two areas (something like a bar magnet which is positive at one end and negative at the other) (Fig. 6.4a). In the case of the heart, the part of the surface which is electrically excited at any one moment will be negative to the unexcited portions. (During depolarization the inside of a cell becomes positive and therefore the outside is negative.) Just as lines of force surround the bar magnet, so lines of electrical potential will surround the heart dipole

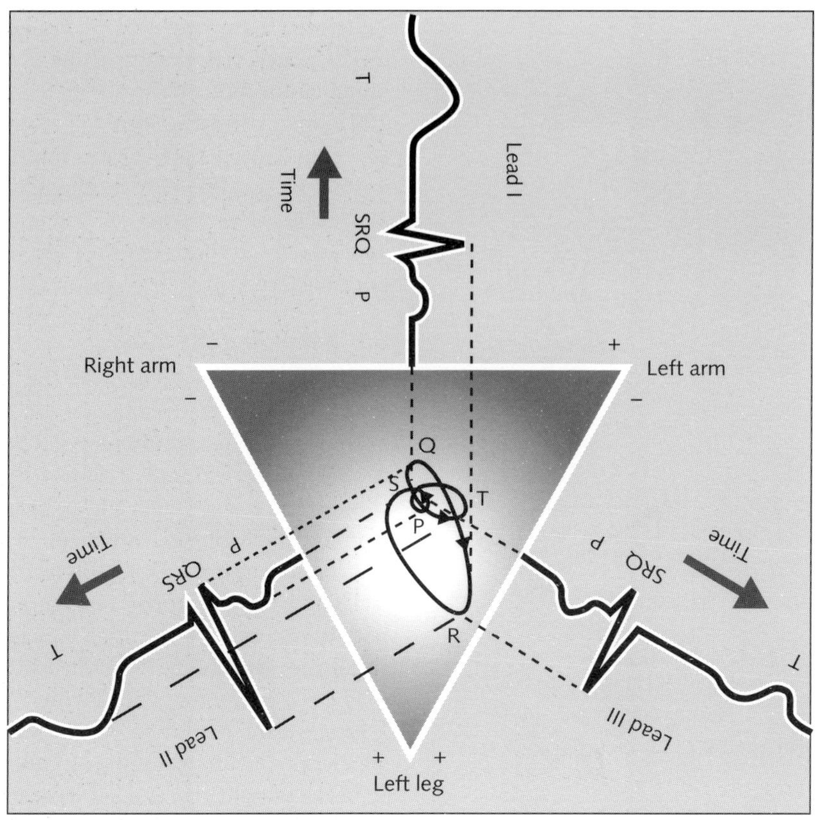

Figure 6.5
Relationship between the changing electrical vectors for the different waves (P–T) and the records in the three standard electrocardiogram (ECG) leads. Each ECG record is the plot against time of the positions of the tip of the cardiac dipole (see Fig. 6.4b) for the various waves. This makes three successive circling sweeps (with pauses between each) giving the form and relative amplitudes of the ECG recordings between the three standard limb leads as shown in Fig. 6.3. (Note that in this projection, two of the records are mirror images of their normal forms.)

during excitation. These extend throughout the body fluids—which, being salt solutions, are good electrical conductors—to the body surface where they can be recorded.

A complication is that as excitation spreads throughout the heart muscle, the orientation of the heart dipole changes. Vectors of electrical potential can be constructed to represent the changing dipole. Like mechanical vectors, these are the resultants of forces which have both magnitude and direction (Fig. 6.4a). These electrical vectors alter in magnitude and direction as excitation proceeds. Figure 6.4b summarizes the way in which the electrical vectors change as the normal excitation wave passes through the myocardium.

Analysis of how the electrical vectors alter at different moments in excitation can explain the different patterns expected from ECG records taken from leads I–III or from chest leads. This is illustrated in Fig. 6.5, where the changes in the vectors for all the waves of the ECG are shown in the centre, and projected to the records obtained from the different limb leads to given both the relative amplitude and different form of these.

If some of the heart muscle becomes damaged, then the usual pattern of vector change will be altered, and alterations in ECG recordings from the different leads can be detected.

As mentioned before the normal ECG trace is at zero potential between the main deflections, i.e. during the P–R and S–T intervals. An elevated or depressed ST segment occurs when part of the myocardium has been damaged. From the damaged, and therefore depolarized region, injury currents will flow to the uninjured muscle and alter the level of the baseline of the ECG or that of the ST segment itself so that this will be raised above the rest of the ECG trace or will sag below it. Figure 6.6a shows these types of altered pattern. Elevation of the ST segment is an indication of acute myocardial damage, usually from a myocardial

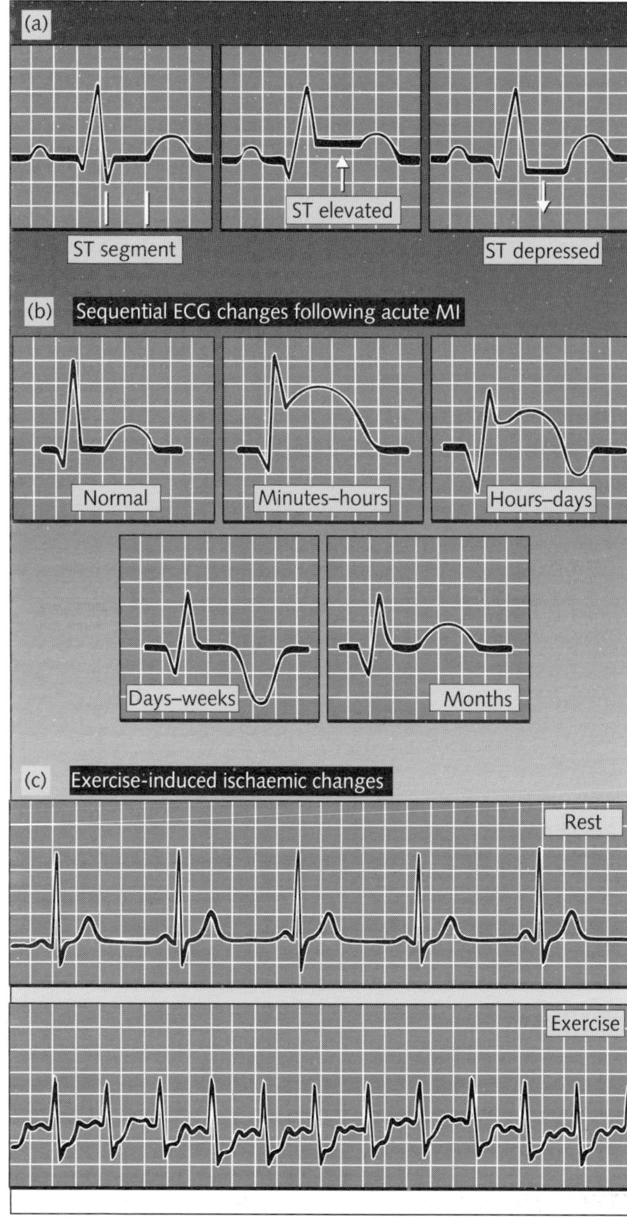

Figure 6.6
(a) Elevated and depressed ST segments, compared with normal electrocardiogram trace. (b) The sequential changes in an electrocardiogram after a myocardial infarction. (c) Depressed ST segment developing in exercise-induced ischaemia.

infarction or MI (often caused by coronary thrombosis, see Chapter 15) or from pericarditis. Figure 6.6b shows the sequential changes in ECG in the acute and recovery phases after an MI.

Depression of the ST segment is usually a sign of ischaemia (restricted blood supply) and in some people occurs only during exercise, while the resting ECG is perfectly normal (Fig. 6.6c).

7 | Arrhythmias: electrophysiological basis

7.1 Introduction

Abnormalities of heart rhythm are known as arrhythmias. They are classified according to two sets of criteria: first, according to their site of origin: atrial, junctional (often combined as supraventricular) or ventricular; second, according to their effect on heart rate—whether they cause an increase in rate (tachycardia) or a decrease in rate (bradycardia). A full clinical classification is given in the next chapter (Table 8.1).

There are two basic causes of arrhythmias which may be present separately or together, these are:

1 malfunction of the conduction system of the heart;

2 abnormal impulse generation—extra excitatory (ectopic) signals occur.

This chapter briefly introduces some of the changes which can lead to arrhythmias. Chapter 8 covers the pharmacology of antiarrhythmic agents while Chapter 9 gives a fuller account of arrhythmias in their clinical context.

7.2 Heart block

Damage to the atrioventricular (AV) node, the only electrical connection between the atria and the ventricles, can lead to heart block. The extent of this can vary depending on the damage to the AV node; it can be partial, when some atrial excitations get through to the ventricles. The block may be quite regular (2:1 or 3:1) and this will show in the ECG as more than one P wave for each QRS-T complex (Fig. 7.1b–d shows ECGs in varying degrees of heartblock; Fig. 7.1a gives a normal ECG for comparison). If the heart block is complete, a latent pacemaker (usually in the Purkinje fibres) will start to generate a rhythm in the ventricles. This will be slower than the normal heart rhythm and now there will be no constant relationship between P waves and QRS-T complexes (Fig. 7.1e).

7.3 Ectopic beats

Latent pacemakers may develop into ectopic foci in the atria or ventricles in the absence of nodal damage and may lead to extrasystoles. Figure 7.1f shows three ventricular extrasystoles (sometimes known as premature ventricular depolarizations) which have arisen from latent pacemakers within the ventricle: the QRS-T complex is much broader than normal because conduction is not occurring down the usual fast conduction pathways. Damage to an area of the myocardium as occurs in myocardial infarction often triggers ectopic impulses in ventricular muscle: damaged cells tend to have depolarized membranes and shorter than normal action potentials — both predisposing factors for ectopic excitation.

7.4 Fibrillation

If multiple ectopic foci develop, discharging asynchronously, the cardiac tissue is said to be fibrillating and does not pump blood. Atrial fibrillation is shown in the ECG record in Fig. 7.1g. QRS complexes can still be identified superimposed on a very irregular baseline, showing that ventricle firing is still coordinated but not regular. Atrial flutter, unlike fibrillation, is regular and probably involves one re-entrant circuit in the lower right atrium (see section 7.6.1. below) rather than the many circuits underlying fibrillations. In atrial flutter the atria usually beat at a frequency of 300/min, but only every second or third impulse is transmitted through the AV node, the others falling within its refractory period, such that the ventricle beats at rate of 150 or 100 beats/min. At the very high rates of atrial fibrillation, only an occasional impulse gets through the AV node, so ventricular excitation occurs at totally irregular intervals, though when it does, QRST complexes can still be recognized.

7.5 Ventricular fibrillation

Ventricular fibrillation (Fig. 7.1h), in which the trace is reduced to oscillations with no sign of QRS-T waves, is a much more serious condition than atrial fibrillation as it results in no cardiac output and thus no perfusion of the brain and other vital organs. It must be treated at once or death will ensue. A defibrillator gives the ventricles a large, brief pulse of electric current, causing every fibre not in the absolute refractory period to discharge. When the fibres regain excitability, coordinated excitation often resumes. Ventricular fibrillation is often preceded by ventricular tachycardia, which is frequently due to an impulse travelling endlessly in a circular movement through the ventricle, resulting in a heart rate often over 180 beats/min (Fig. 7.1i).

Further details of these and related conditions and their clinical manifestations are given in Chapter 9 and more ECGs are shown in Figs 9.1 and 9.2.

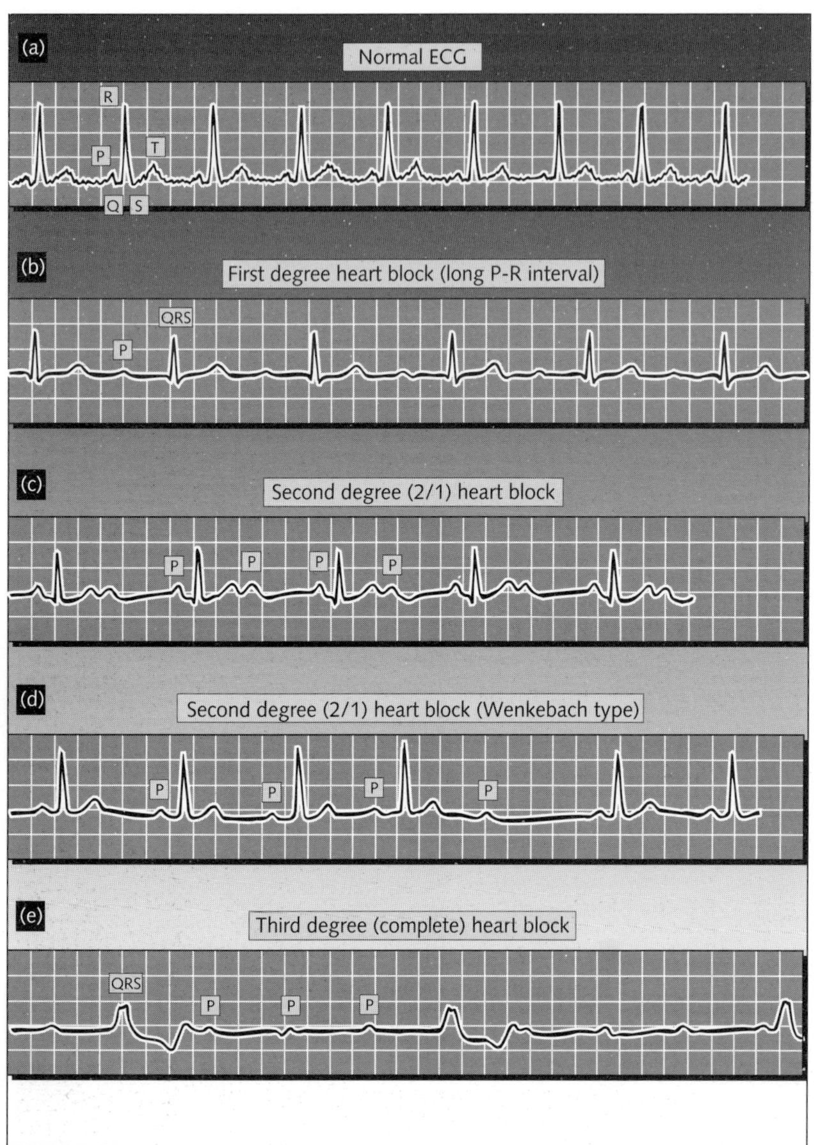

Figure 7.1
(a) Normal electrocardiogram. (b) First degree heart block. There is a constant but abnormally long PR interval (>200 ms) but all beats are conducted. (c) Second degree heart block (Mobitz type II). There is a constant PR interval but every second P wave is not conducted, hence 2/1 block. (d) Second degree heart block (Wenkebach type). There is progressive lengthening of the PR interval, one non-conducted beat and then the next beat has a shorter PR interval. (e) Third degree (complete) heart block. There is no relationship between P waves and the broad QRS complexes.

7.6 Electrophysiological basis of arrhythmia

This section introduces the electrophysiological abnormalities which can precipitate ventricular tachycardia and fibrillation. They are illustrated and summarized in Fig. 7.5 later in this chapter.

7.6.1 Re-entry

One reason for the development of arrhythmias is unequal conduction velocities in two branches of the cardiac muscle network which can lead to what is known as re-entry. In Fig. 7.2, the impulse arriving at point S will normally travel down the two branches, L and R, at the same speed so that at point C it will be extinguished as each impulse encounters membrane refractory from the passage of the other. If the impulse travels more slowly down branch R than down branch L, then the faster-travelling impulse may be able to travel from L, up branch R from the bottom and re-enter tissue already excited. For this to occur unidirectional block must occur at point R (Fig. 7.2d). This could arise, for example, if conduction were slowed in branch R so that the antegrade impulse arrived during the refractory period from a previous excitation and so was extinguished. The retrograde impulse, travel-

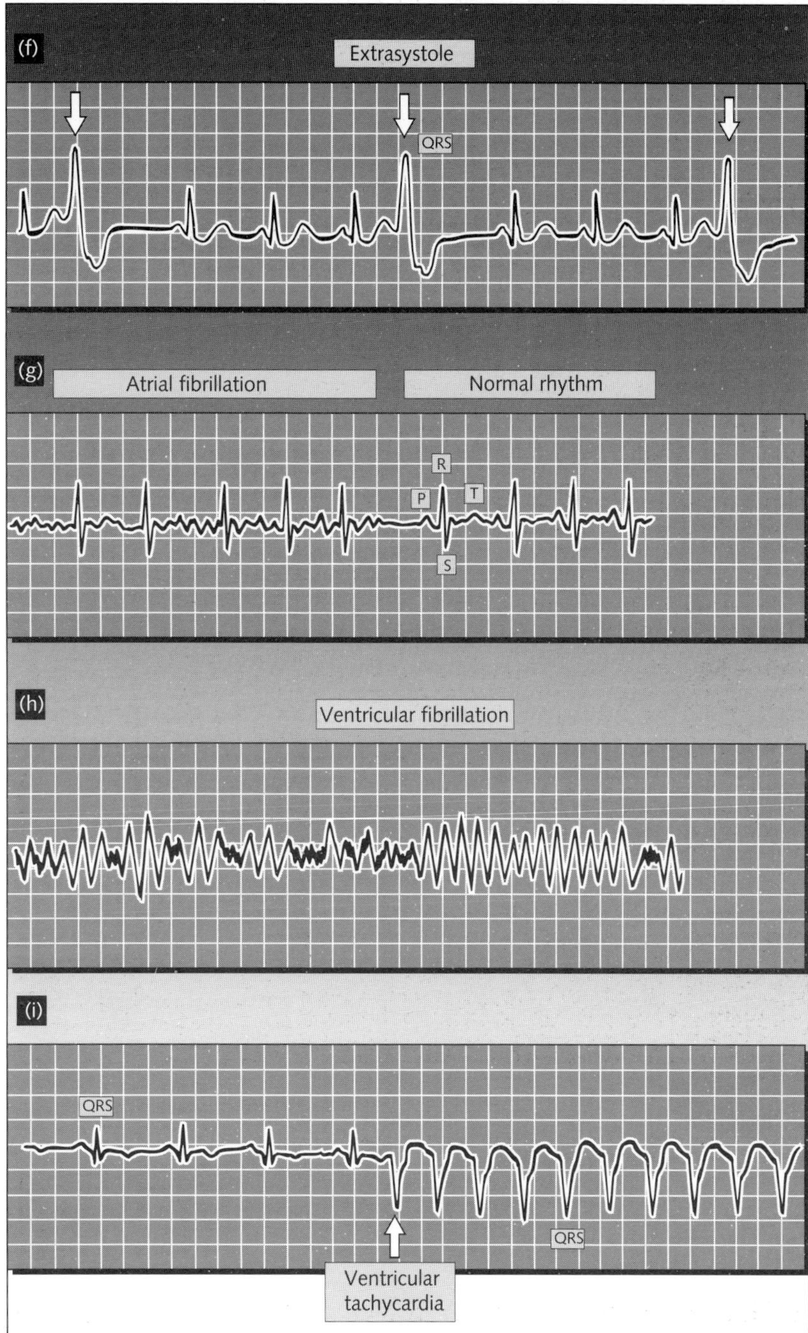

Figure 7.1
(*Continued.*) (f) Ventricular extrasystoles (arrowed). (g) Atrial fibrillation, with a chaotic baseline indicating continual, but erratic, atrial activity and an irregular ventricular response reflecting random bombardment of the atrioventricular node with impulses. Halfway through this trace normal sinus rhythm is restored. (h) Ventricular fibrillation; entirely erratic QRS behaviour. (i) Ventricular tachycardia. Tachycardia starts halfway through this trace. Grid squares = 200 ms and 0.5 mV in all records. (Parts (a–e) courtesy of Dr C.J. Plummer, Freeman Hospital, Newcastle upon Tyne.)

ling via the longer pathway, would arrive later when the refractory period was over. Once established, such loops can become self-perpetuating and lead to fibrillation.

Re-entry loops can be large or small and include all types of cardiac muscle. When there is an extra electrical pathway outside the AV node making such a loop, self-perpetuating (circus) excitation can develop between the atria and ventricles (e.g. via the bundle of Kent in the Wolff–Parkinson–White syndrome) giving episodes of paroxysmal tachycardia in which the ventricles beat at 200/min or more.

The slow conduction velocity which leads to re-entry can itself arise from a variety of causes. One of the most common is localized hyperkalaemia (raised external potassium con-

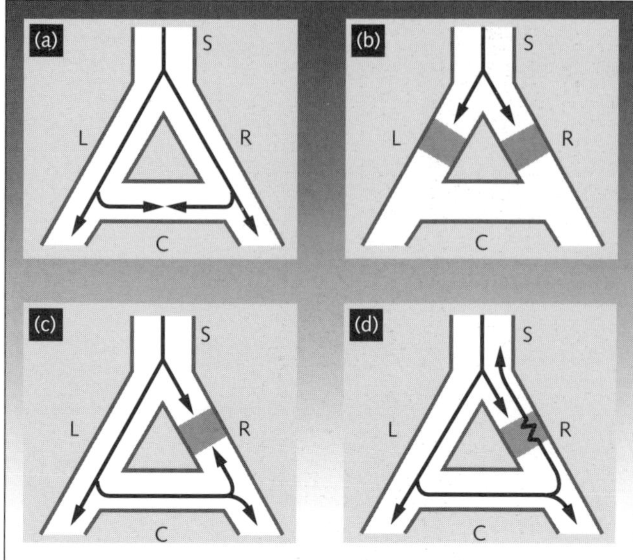

Figure 7.2
The way in which unidirectional block can lead to re-entry. (a) Excitation passing down a single bundle of cardiac muscle will, when this divides, continue down the two branches, L and R. On entering the connecting bundle (C) it will not be able to travel beyond the zone of collision as beyond that the tissue will be refractory to further excitation. (b) Excitation is blocked in both L and R branches. (c) Bi-directional block in branch R. (d) Unidirectional block in branch R; this could occur if the tissue at the top of branch R has had time to recover from refractoriness before the retrograde excitation reaches it via L and C.

centration) which will cause depolarization of cell membranes with consequent inactivation of some of the fast sodium channels and shorter action potentials with more slowly rising upstrokes, dependent largely on inward calcium current, $i_{Ca,L}$, which are consequently more slowly conducted. (The effects of raised external potassium on the ventricular action potential are shown in Fig. 14.1.) The localized hyperkalaemia itself often arises from cellular damage in ischaemic tissue.

Scarred areas of heart muscle which remain after a myocardial infarction has occurred can form foci for re-entry circuits which can lead to ventricular tachycardias, with the risk of ventricular fibrillation (see further discussion of this in Chapter 9). Here, disrupted electrical coupling between cells in the scar region may lead to slowed conduction and hence re-entry circuits.

7.6.2 After-depolarizations

Delayed after-depolarizations

Inward membrane currents can sometimes trigger arrhythmias. Transient inward current is net inward current developed during sodium/calcium exchange across the cardiac membrane (see also Chapter 4). When cardiac cells are overloaded with calcium these inward currents assume an intermittent oscillatory mode and can become dangerously large, resulting in delayed after-depolarizations or DADs which may trigger extrasystoles (Fig. 7.3a).

Early after-depolarizations

In contrast to DADs, which are depolarizations from the resting potential, occurring after depolarization is complete, early after-depolarizations (EADs) occur *before* repolarization is complete, prolonging the plateau of the action potential in an oscillatory manner (Fig. 7.3b). Unlike DADs, which are exacerbated by tachycardia, EADs diminish in tachycar-

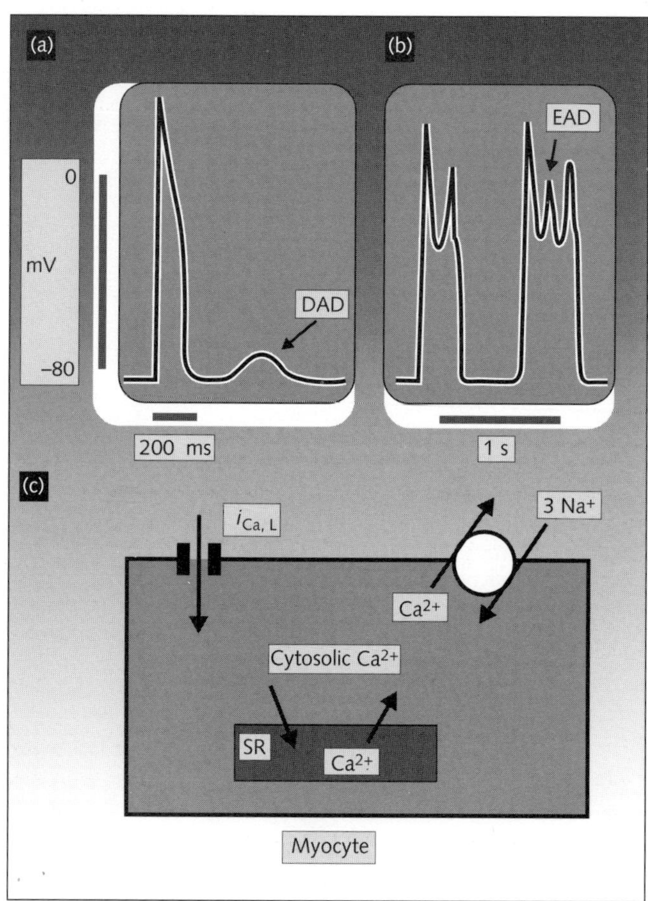

Figure 7.3
(a) and (b) After-depolarizations in guinea-pig ventricular cells; (a) a delayed after-depolarization (DAD); (b) early after-depolarizations (EADs); (c) Ca^{2+} movements underlying DADs: increased cytosolic Ca^{2+} levels cause pulses of Ca^{2+} release from the sarcoplasmic reticulum (SR) which in turn lead to bursts of Na^+/Ca^{2+} exchange activity giving inward current and hence membrane depolarizations (DADs).

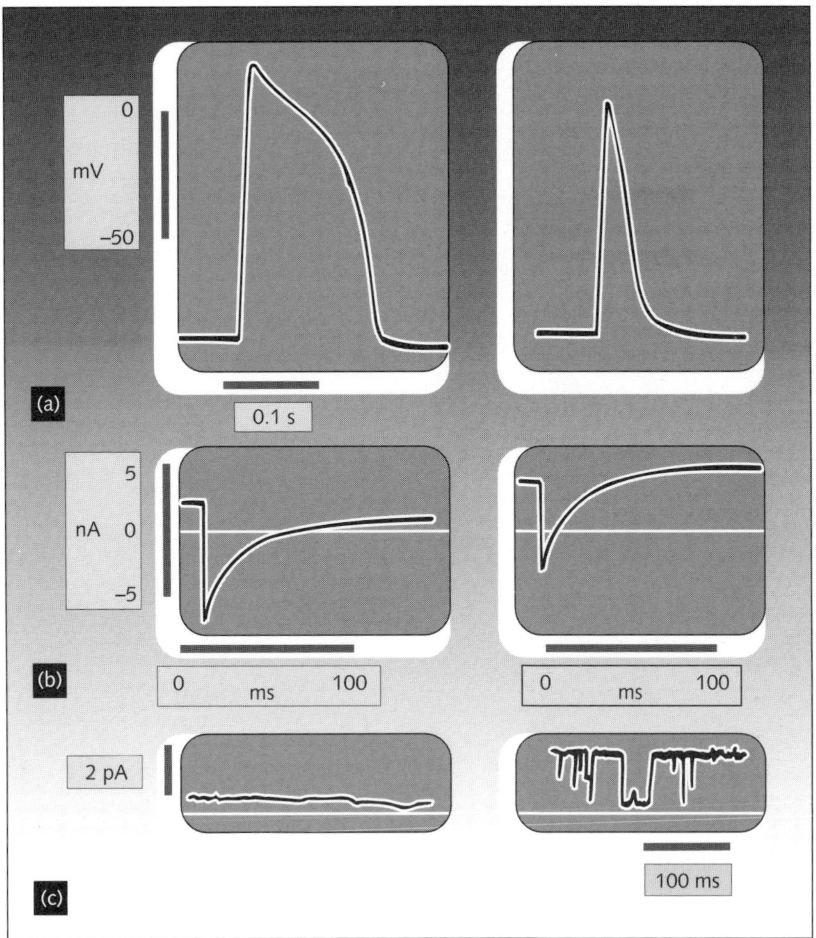

Figure 7.4
Adenosine triphosphate (ATP)-sensitive potassium channels. (a) Action potentials recorded from guinea-pig papillary muscle in normal Tyrode solution (left) and after removal of oxygen and glucose (right). As ATP levels fall, ATP-sensitive potassium channels will open and shorten the action potential. (b) Currents recorded from a guinea-pig ventricular myocyte in response to a voltage clamp step from −40 to +12 mV in normal Tyrode solution (left) and, on the right, in the presence of 0.2 mmol/l DNP (a metabolic blocker). Opening of ATP-sensitive channels as ATP levels fall contributes a large outward current causing the outward (upscreen) shift in the current record in DNP. (c) Single channel recording from an inside-out patch of guinea-pig ventricular myocyte membrane showing openings of ATP-sensitive K^+ channels when (righthand panel) 0.2 mM DNP was applied. (Courtesy of Dr J. Vereecke, Catholic University of Leuven.)

dia. Bradycardia or conditions which prolong the action potential (hypokalaemia, as can result from diuretic therapy, or treatment with antiarrhythmic drugs which prolong the QT interval) can lead to EADs and the associated arrhythmia known as torsade de pointes (see Fig. 9.2e and Chapter 9). It is suggested that EADs result from a 'window' calcium current: as the membrane repolarizes, it passes through a voltage range where calcium channels reopen and give rise to an extra depolarization.

7.6.3 Hypoxia: adenosine triphosphate-sensitive potassium channels

Potassium channels which are opened by a fall in ATP concentration are found in many types of cell. They were first observed in cardiac (ventricular) cells in 1983 by Professor A. Noma. The outward current that will flow through such channels radically shortens the action potential (Fig. 7.4). Such channels seem to be important in the response to hypoxic conditions such as ischaemia. It is suggested that since such short action potentials lead to reduced contractions, the ischaemic muscle will be spared until conditions improve, but such shortening of the action potential can also be pro-arrhythmic.

7.6.4 Catecholamines

Catecholamines can trigger arrhythmias (see also Chapters 8

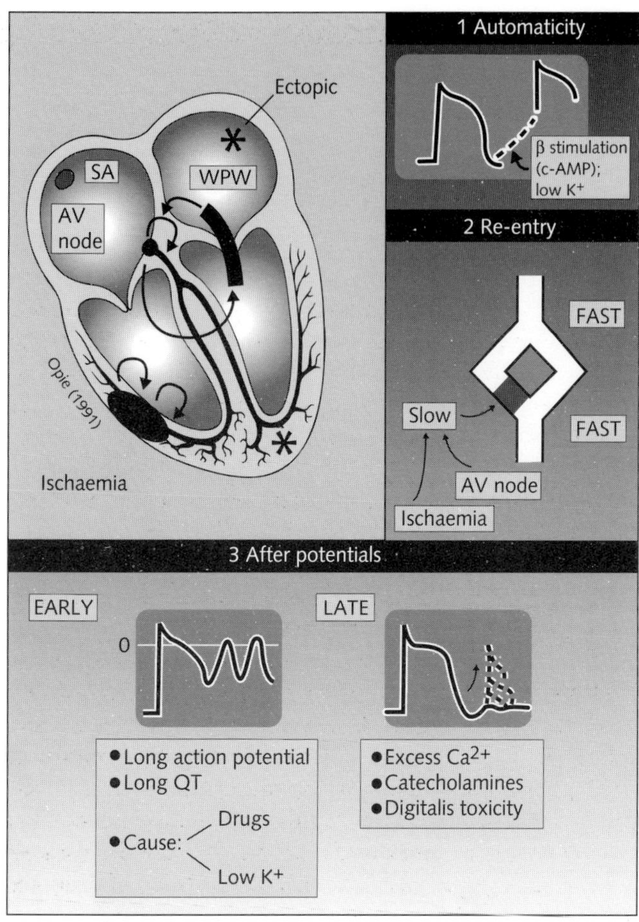

Figure 7.5
Summary of causes of arrhythmia. SA, sinoatrial node; WPW, Wolff–Parkinson–White accessory pathway. (Redrawn with permission from Opie, L.H. (1991) *The Heart. Physiology and Metabolism*, 2nd edn. Raven Press, New York.)

and 9). One way in which they do so appears to be by inducing an inward chloride current which increases the excitability of ventricular cells.

Figure 7.5 summarizes the various factors which can lead to ventricular fibrillation.

8 Antiarrhythmic drugs

8.1 Introduction

The control of arrhythmia by antiarrhythmic agents is one of the most complicated and challenging problems of medical practice. While the general approach to therapy still remains empirical, some novel rational drug treatments are being investigated. There remain, however, considerable problems and these were recently highlighted when an extensive clinical trial (the CAST trial) revealed potentially lethal side-effects of antiarrhythmic drugs in widespread use. Encainide and flecainide, for example, were reported to cause a two- to threefold increase in mortality compared to placebo when given to patients who had had a myocardial infarction (see section 8.4 for a summary of the outcome of recent antiarrhythmic trials).

8.2 Classification of antiarrhythmic drugs

Antiarrhythmic agents were originally classified by Vaughan Williams on the basis of their predominant antiarrhythmic action (Table 8.1). This classification was intended to categorize the antiarrhythmic actions of drugs and not the drugs themselves so that drugs within a single class are not necessarily similar in chemical structure. A patient may therefore respond to one drug within a single class, but not to another.

Another classification (the Sicilian Gambit, so called because it originated at a meeting held in Taormina, Sicily, in 1990) groups antiarrhythmic drugs according to their site of action: sodium channel, β-receptor, Na/K pump, etc. This has not yet, however, been generally adopted and the following account will be based on the more widely used Vaughan Williams classification.

On looking at a summary of a range of antiarrhythmic agents together with their antiarrhythmic actions (such as is given in Table 8.2 later in this chapter) it is apparent that a given compound can exhibit antiarrhythmic action of several classes and it is often unclear which of these actions is responsible for suppression of arrhythmia in a given patient. It can indeed be the multiple actions themselves which are responsible for a high degree of antiarrhythmic efficiency, as in the case of amiodarone.

8.3 Antiarrhythmic agents

8.3.1 Class I

The early observation that atrial fibrillation occurring in patients with malaria would sometimes be cured when they were treated with the quinine-containing cinchona bark was followed up by Wenckebach, who in 1914 reported on the effects of quinine alkaloids in certain cardiac arrhythmias. Soon after this it was found that quinidine, a *d*-isomer of quinine, was the most effective of these drugs for treating atrial fibrillation.

Class I antiarrhythmic drugs exert their action by blocking cardiac sodium channels (Fig. 8.1). This reduces the excitability in those parts of the heart (the non-nodal regions) where the inward sodium current plays an important role in propagation of the cardiac action potential.

The sodium channel-blocking action of class I compounds is identical to that of local anaesthetics. The non-ionized lipid-soluble form of the drug penetrates the cell membrane and enters the cell interior. Once inside the cell a proportion of drug molecules, depending on their pK_a, are protonated and in this form they interact with the sodium channel. This local anaesthetic action is also shown by class I agents in nervous tissue, although higher concentrations of drug are required for this than for the antiarrhythmic actions.

Sodium channels have three states: open, closed and inactivated (refractory). Class I antiarrhythmic agents can only bind to the channel while it is open and once bound they serve to stabilize its inactivated state. Thus they are more effective at blocking frequently occurring action potentials—a phenomenon known as use-dependent block. This can be shown experimentally in myocardial preparations which can be electrically stimulated at different frequencies.

Class I antiarrhythmic agents can be subclassified according to the kinetics of their binding and unbinding to the sodium channel.

- Class Ia, e.g. quinidine, procainamide and disopyramide (Fig. 8.1). These agents are the earliest examples of class I antiarrhythmic agents (see above) and represent the benchmark to which agents falling into Class Ib and Ic are compared. Their properties fall midway between those of these latter subclasses (see below). They are often used for tachycardias of atrial or nodal origin (supraventricular tachycardias), though they are also active on ventricular tissue.
- Class Ib drugs, e.g. lignocaine, mexiletine and tocainide (Fig. 8.1). These drugs associate and dissociate rapidly. Thus they bind to sodium channels during the upstroke (phase 0) of the action potential, having little effect on the rate of rise

Table 8.1
The Vaughan Williams classification of antiarrhythmic actions of drugs and their adverse cardiac effects.

Class	Common name	Action	Prototypes	Adverse effects
I	Na-channel blockers	Na-channel block	Lignocaine Procainamide	Proarrhythmic effect Negative inotropic effect (rate-dependent)
II	β-blockers	Antagonism of sympathetic nervous stimulation and circulating catecholamines	Propranolol	Sinus bradycardia Atrioventricular block Depression of left ventricular function
III	K-channel blockers	Increased refractoriness	Amiodarone Bretylium	Sinus bradycardia Torsade de Pointes
IV	Ca^{2+}-channel blockers (antagonists)	Prevention of Ca^{2+} entry	Verapamil Nifedipine	Atrioventricular block Negative ionotropy
V*	Miscellaneous	Miscellaneous	Alinidine Digoxin (as an antiarrhythmic)	Sinus bradycardia

* Class V drugs not always recognized as a coherent group.

but leaving many of the channels unavailable for further activation by the time the action potential reaches its peak. They then dissociate for the next action potential if the cardiac rhythm is normal but will prevent premature beats, because the sodium channels will still be unavailable when these might occur. These agents also bind selectively to refractory sodium channels, e.g. those present in ischaemic regions where the cells are depolarized. This subclass is thus particularly useful in the control of ventricular arrhythmias which follow myocardial infarctions.

- Class Ic: flecainide and encainide (Fig. 8.1). Drugs in this subclass associate and dissociate much more slowly than those of class Ia. They therefore cause a steady-state level of sodium channel block that does not vary appreciably during the cardiac cycle and that causes a general reduction in excitability. Thus they will suppress re-entrant rhythms which depend on unidirectional or intermittent conduction pathways. They show only a marginal preference for refractory channels and are therefore of limited use in a damaged or ischaemic myocardium. They are used for life-threatening ventricular tachycardias, but with great caution after the results of the CAST trial (see section 8.4 below).

Class I antiarrhythmics are generally metabolized by the liver and should not be given in hepatic impairment. Side-effects associated with their action include hypotension, confusion and convulsions.

8.3.2 Class II antiarrhythmic agents (β-blockers)

It has been known for a number of years that cardiac arrhythmias can be induced or exacerbated by stress or emotion. Sympathetic stimulation or the presence of catecholamines is known to encourage arrhythmia formation. Experimentally induced arrhythmias may be substantially reduced by thoracic sympathectomy and cardiac denervation, while stellate ganglion stimulation increases sensitivity to arrhythmias. Furthermore, there is a close association between palpitation, tachycardia and arrhythmia in patients with phaeochromocytoma (an adrenaline-secreting tumour). Paradoxically, however, at times of extreme stress or emotion vagal activity can predominate, leading to bradycardia rather than tachycardia.

Sympathetic transmitters interact with β-adrenoreceptors and via activation of adenylate cyclase raise intracellular cyclic adenosine monophosphate (cAMP). This in turn opens (through phosphorylation via protein kinase A) calcium channels enhancing the inward calcium current, $i_{Ca,L}$. The rates of sinoatrial (SA) node discharge and the rate of conduction in SA and atrioventricular (AV) nodal tissue are both increased when $i_{Ca,L}$ increases. β-Agonists can also make ventricular cells more excitable, partly by the increase in $i_{Ca,L}$ they cause and also by inducing an inward current carried by chloride ions (see Chapter 14). β-Blockers are successfully used to reduce the occurrence of ventricular arrhythmias after myocardial infarctions, which are partly the result of increased sympathetic activity. They are also used to slow conduction within the AV node and so to reduce the ventricular rate in supraventricular tachycardias.

Class II drugs are illustrated in Fig. 8.2. The main ones now used for arrhythmias (and for hypertension and angina) are metoprolol and atenolol. Metoprolol is a class II agent

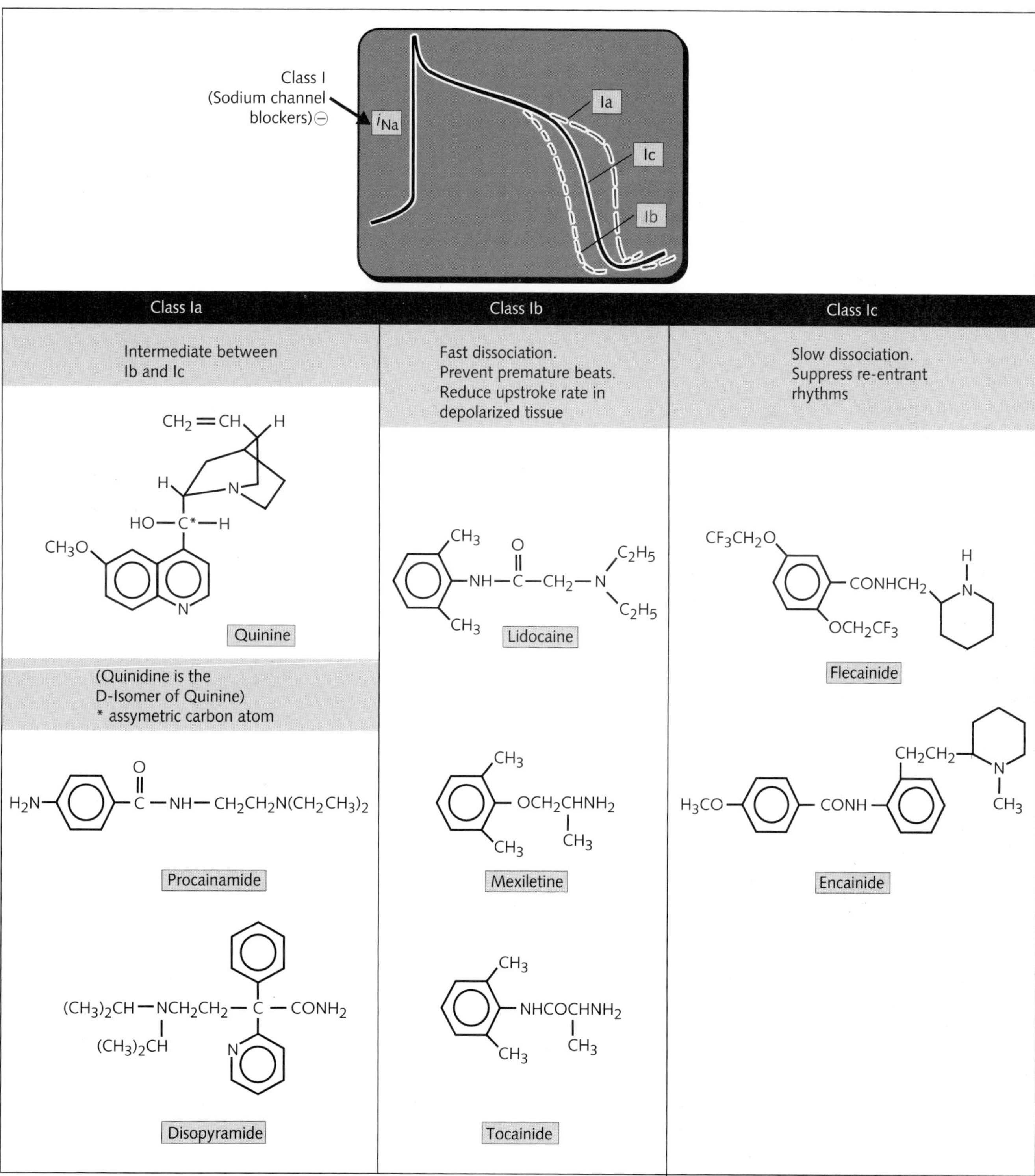

Figure 8.1
Class I antiarrhythmic drugs. Used for supraventricular tachycardias, control of post-infarction ventricular arrhythmias and life threatening ventricular tachycardias. (Top) Points of action, illustrated on a Purkinje fibre action potential. The effects on action potential duration of the three subclasses are indicated. (Bottom) Main drugs, with structures in the subclasses Ia, Ib and Ic.

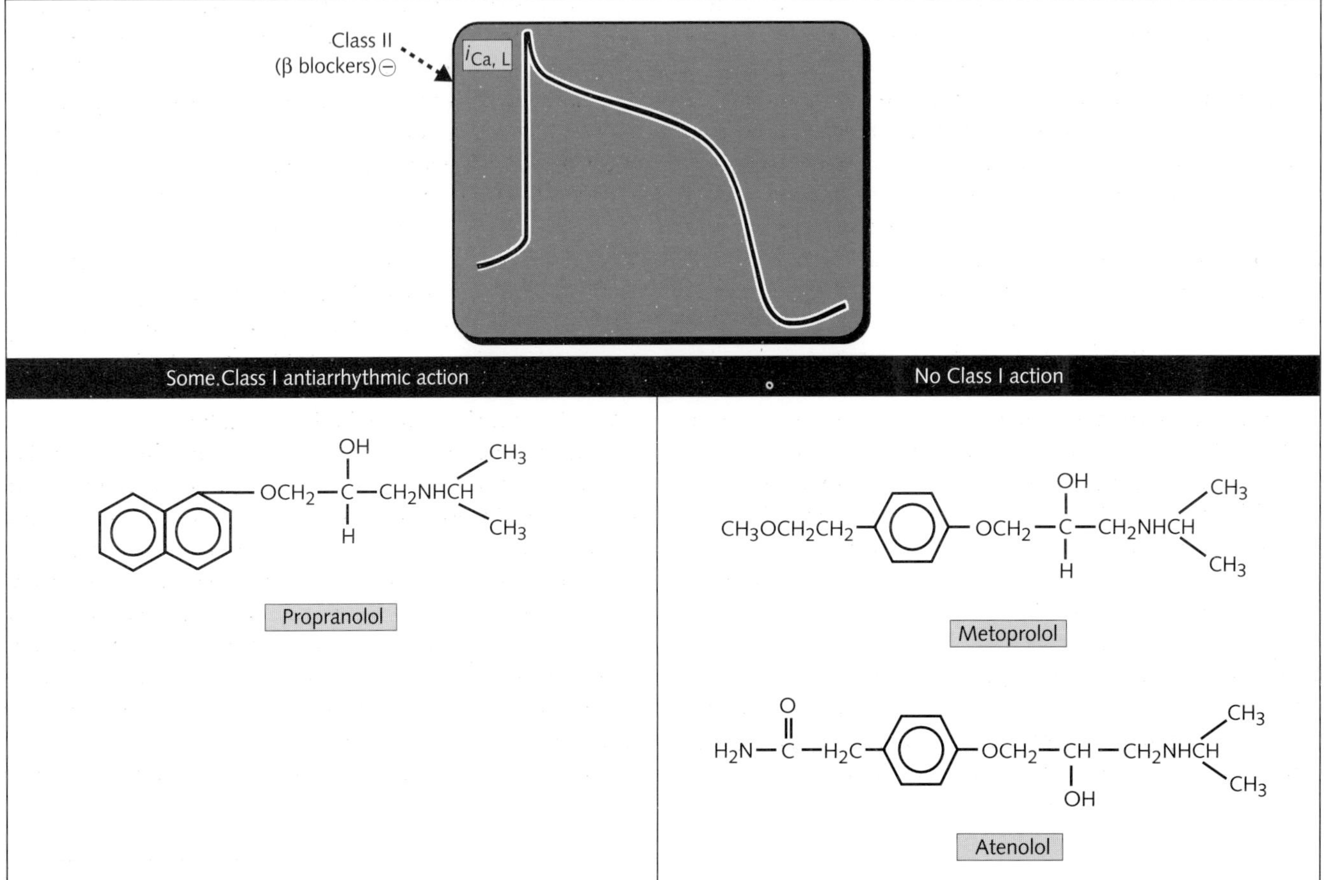

Figure 8.2
Class II antiarrhythmic drugs. Used for the prevention of post-infarction arrhythmias and supraventricular tachycardias. (Top) Point of action, illustrated on a Purkinje fibre action potential. (Bottom) Main drugs in class II, with structures.

which does not exhibit class I activity. Propranolol was the first β-blocker to be introduced into therapy (in 1965). In addition to class II actions it also shows some class I antiarrhythmic effects (local anaesthetic properties). It is now used in the treatment of some conditions such as phaeochromocytoma (an adrenaline/noradrenaline secreting tumour of adrenal medullary tissue) and for thyrotoxicosis.

While virtually all other antiarrhythmic agents in large multicentre trials have been shown either to have no impact on mortality or indeed are associated with an excess mortality (see below), β-blockers have been shown to reduce mortality, particularly by reducing sudden cardiac death after a heart attack. In addition to their use as antiarrhythmic agents, β-blockers are useful in the treatment of ischaemic heart disease (Chapter 16).

8.3.3 Class III antiarrhythmic agents

Class III antiarrhythmic agents induce a prolongation of the action potential which markedly increases the refractory period of the myocardium. The exact mechanism of action of class III agents is not fully understood, although it is likely to be due to block of potassium channels. It is not certain which potassium current is inhibited by class III agents: the delayed rectifier, i_K, the inward rectifier, i_{K1} and the transient outward current, i_{to}, may all be affected. (For an account of the properties of these currents and their role in cardiac action potentials, see Chapter 4).

Since i_K plays a part in initiating repolarization, block of this current can be expected to increase the duration of the action potential plateau and prolong the refractory period. Support for this idea comes from its converse: opening of adenosine triphosphate (ATP)-sensitive potassium channels when ATP levels fall in, for example, ischaemic conditions (see Chapter 7 and Fig. 7.4) tends to reduce the refractory period of myocardial tissue. A shorter refractory period gives more opportunity for ectopic excitation to establish excitatory circuits (see Chapter 7) and ischaemia with associated reduction of refractory period does lead to an arrhythmogenic state, at least in animal models.

The most notable class III agents are amiodarone and the dextro (*d*) isomer of sotalol (Fig. 8.3). Amiodarone, which is much used clinically in intensive care situations, prolongs action potential duration and increases refractoriness. This is presumably by a blocking effect on potassium channels but it has not been conclusively proven that this action underlies its clinical effectiveness or which potassium channel(s) is(are) chiefly involved. Sotalol has two isomers: *d*, which only has class III action and *l*, which is also a powerful β-blocker. *d*-Sotalol tends to prolong action potential duration and increases the refractory period of the ventricles *in vivo* without affecting conduction velocity in normal or ischaemic tissue. Recent evidence suggests this action, like that of other class III agents, is due to potassium current inhibition. A recent clinical trial (the SWORD or survival with oral *d*-sotalol trial) of *d*-sotalol has, however, shown that in some situations it increases rather than decreases mortality.

8.3.4 Class IV antiarrhythmic agents (calcium antagonists)

The characteristic action of drugs in this category is inhibition of calcium movement through voltage-activated, L-type calcium channels (Chapter 16). When used as antiarrhythmic agents class IV drugs act primarily on the SA and AV nodes, i.e. where the action potential upstroke depends on $i_{Ca,L}$. This contrasts with class I antiarrhythmic drugs, which affect the fast sodium channel and which act, therefore, predominantly on the non-nodal regions of the heart. The action of class IV agents therefore results in a slowing of conduction and prolongation of refractory period in nodal tissue. Conduction through ischaemic regions is also slowed: in ischaemia, the cell membranes tend to be depolarized and this will inactivate some of the Na^+ channels, giving action potentials with upstrokes more dependent on the slower $i_{Ca,L}$ (see Chapter 14), and which are therefore more slowly conducted. (These are sometimes known as slow responses.) Class IV antiarrhythmics will slow them further.

Calcium blockers are used to control the ventricular response rate in supraventricular tachycardias such as atrial fibrillation. Key examples of this class used as antiarrhythmics are verapamil and diltiazem (Fig. 8.4). Verapamil was the first calcium antagonist to be introduced and is relatively selective for cardiac calcium channels. Diltiazem is less specific: it also relaxes smooth muscle, thereby inducing hypotension. Nifedipine and related drugs work predominantly on vascular smooth muscle and are used to treat hypertension (see Chapter 16).

A consequence of the reduction in inward calcium current

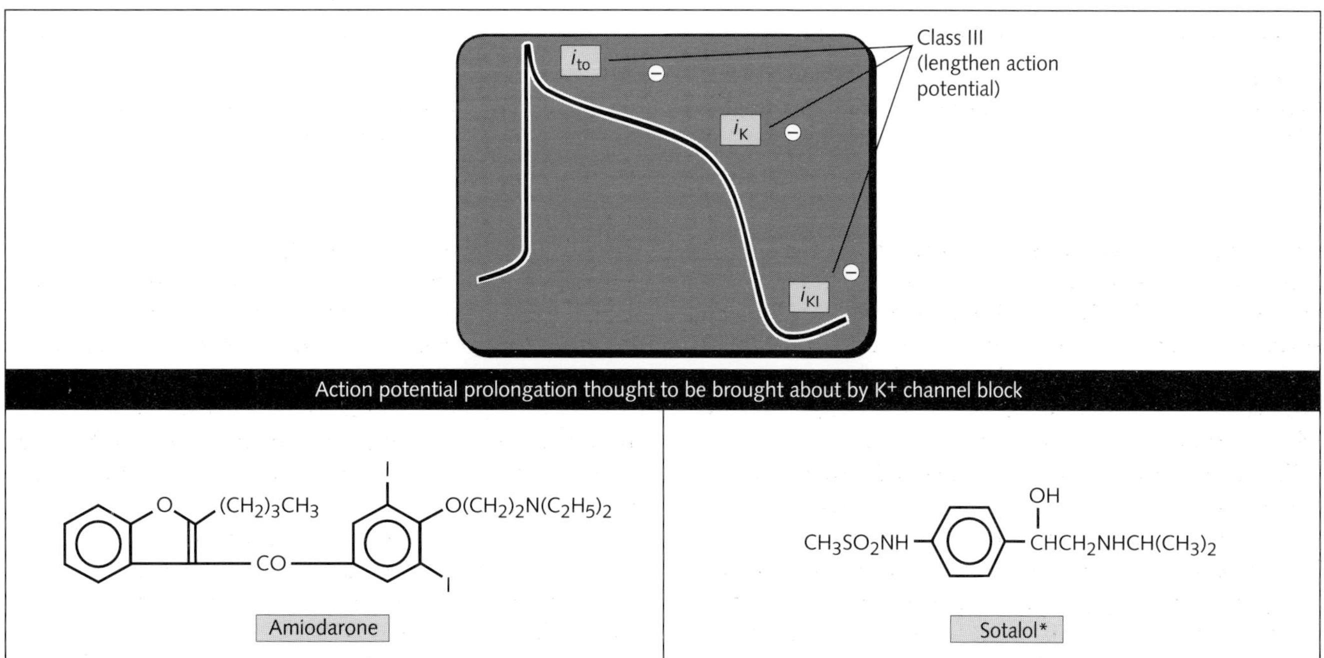

Figure 8.3
Class III antiarrhythmic drugs. Used for tachycardias. (Top) Points of action, illustrated on a Purkinje fibre action potential. (Bottom) Main drugs in class III, with structures.

* To be used with caution after recent clinical trial.

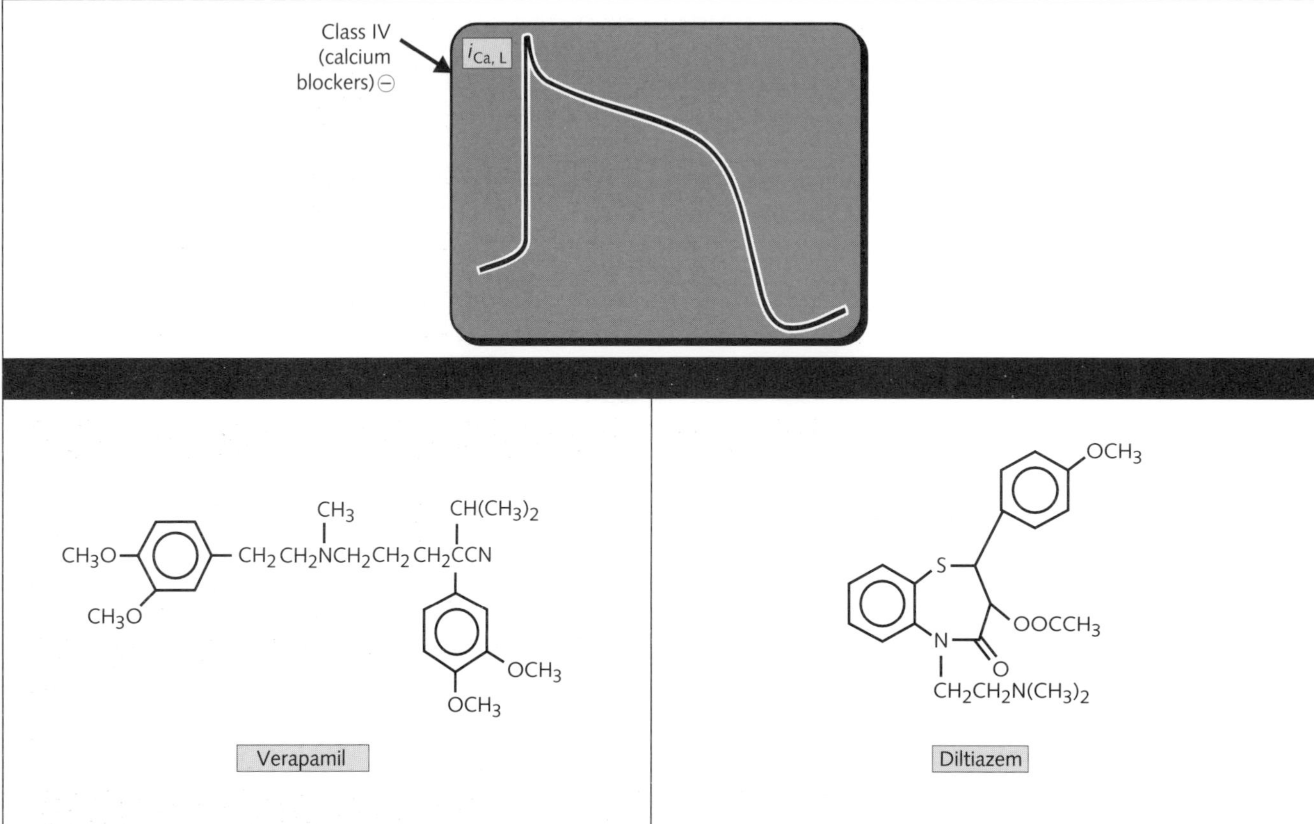

Figure 8.4
Class IV antiarrhythmic drugs. Used for supraventricular tachycardias. (Top) Point of action, illustrated on a Purkinje fibre action potential. (Bottom) Main drugs in class IV, with structures.

brought about by class IV drugs is a shortening of the plateau phase of the myocardial action potential. Shorter action potentials and the slower conduction velocity which also results from calcium current reduction can both be proarrhythmic factors in the ventricle. The shortened action potentials will also lead to weaker contractions.

In addition to the treatment of arrhythmia, calcium antagonists are also useful in the treatment of ischaemic heart disease (Chapter 16).

8.3.5 Class V (miscellaneous) antiarrhythmic agents

The action of agents assigned to this group is not entirely clear and the group is miscellaneous. Examples of drugs which fall into this category are given below and in Fig. 8.5.

- Digoxin. A cardiac glycoside, digoxin, is used therapeutically for the treatment of heart failure on account of its positive inotropic action (Chapter 18). It is used in atrial fibrillation because it acts within the central nervous system to increase vagal parasympathetic activity (see Chapter 12), thus slowing conduction within the AV node and hence reducing the high ventricular rate which results from atrial fibrillation. This action does not abolish the fibrillation but ameliorates its effect.
- Adenosine. Adenosine and ATP act via purinergic P_2 and P_1 receptors, respectively. These agents are useful for the treatment of supraventricular tachycardias. It is important to note that the effects of ATP are due to its rapid metabolism in the plasma to adenosine. In cardiac nodal tissue stimulation of P_1 receptors results in activation of G-protein-coupled potassium channels which cause hyperpolarization. The potassium channels activated by adenosine are similar to those regulated by acetylcholine as a consequence of parasympathetic nervous stimulation. Stimulation of these receptors reduces automaticity and conduction, causing sinus bradycardia and AV block.
- Alinidine. This agent, a derivative of the α-adrenoceptor agonist clonidine, prolongs action potential duration. *In*

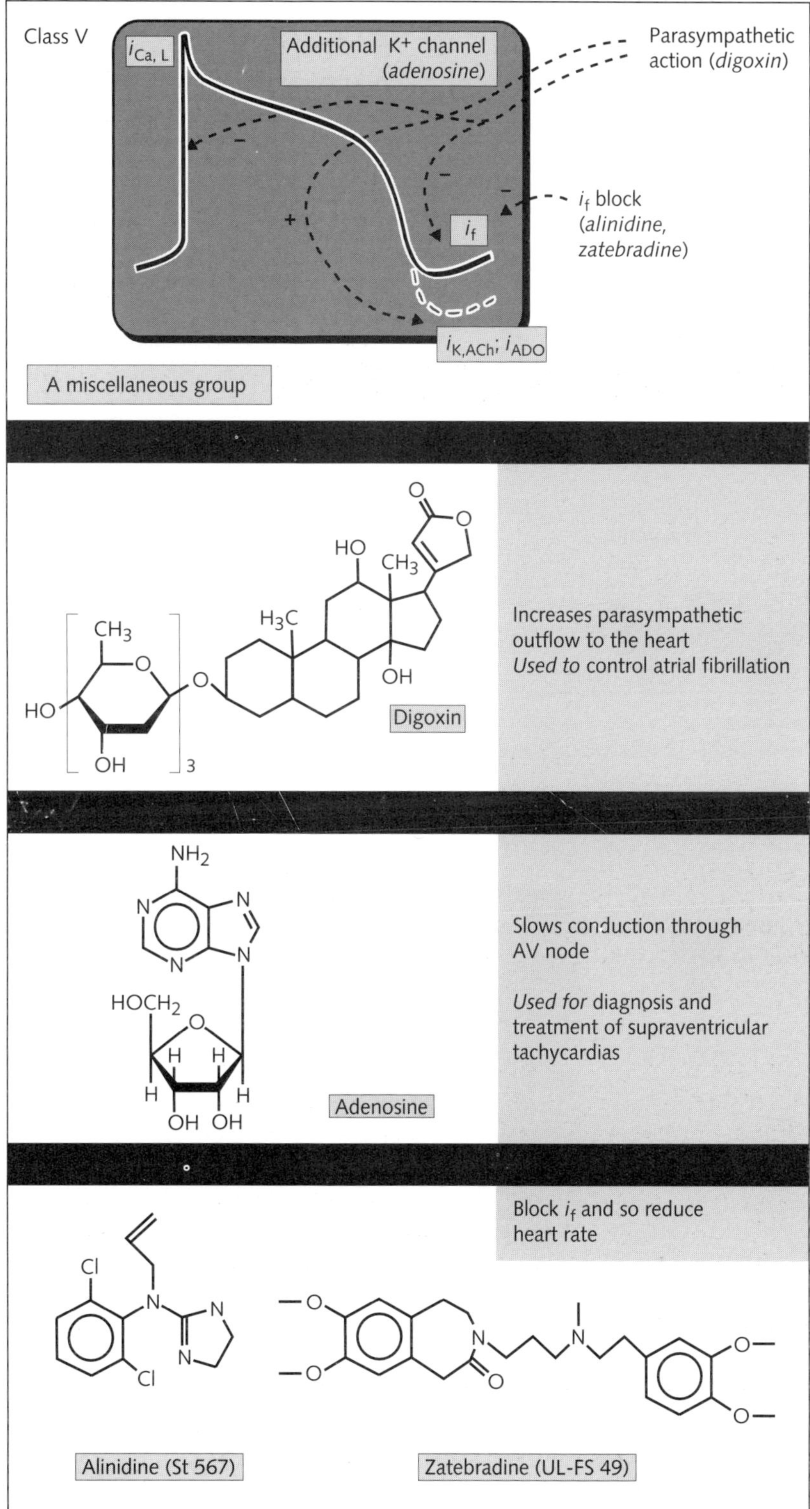

Figure 8.5
'Class V' antiarrhythmic drugs.
(Top) Points of action of digoxin (as an antiarrhythmic), adenosine and of i_f blockers. For clarity and uniformity, the actions of this miscellaneous group are illustrated on a Purkinje fibre action potential rather than on the supraventricular sites where they act clinically. Digoxin and adenosine exert their antiarrhythmic actions primarily on the atrioventricular node where the additional K^+ channels they activate will cause considerable hyperpolarization and slowing. (Below) Drugs in class V, with structures.

Table 8.2
Antiarrhythmic actions.

Class	Examples	Mechanism	Cardiac effects				
			MRD	APD	ERP	AV conduction	Contraction
Ia	Quinidine	Block of Na channels	↓↓	↑	↑	↓↓	↓
	Procainamide		↓↓	↑	↑	↓↓	↓
	Disopyramide		↓↓	↑	↑	↓↓	↓↓↓
Ib	Lignocaine	Block of Na channels (fast dissociation)	↓↓↓*	↓	↑↑	—	—
	Mexiletine		↓↓↓*	↓	↑↑	—	—
	Tocainide		↓↓↓*	↓	↑↑	↓	—
Ic	Flecainide	Block of Na channels (slow dissociation)	↓↓↓	—	—	↓↓	↓↓
	Encainide		↓↓↓	—	—	↓↓	↓↓
II	Propranolol	β-Adrenoceptor antagonism	—	—	—	— or ↓	↓↓
	Metoprolol		—	—	—		↓↓
III	Amiodarone	Not known	—	↑↑↑	↑↑↑	↓	↑
IV	Verapamil	Calcium channel block	—	↓↓	—	↓↓	↓↓↓
	Diltiazem		—	↓	—	↓	

MRD, Maximum rate of depolarization; APD, action potential duration; ERP, effective refractory period; AV, atrioventricular.
* Reduced only in depolarized cells.

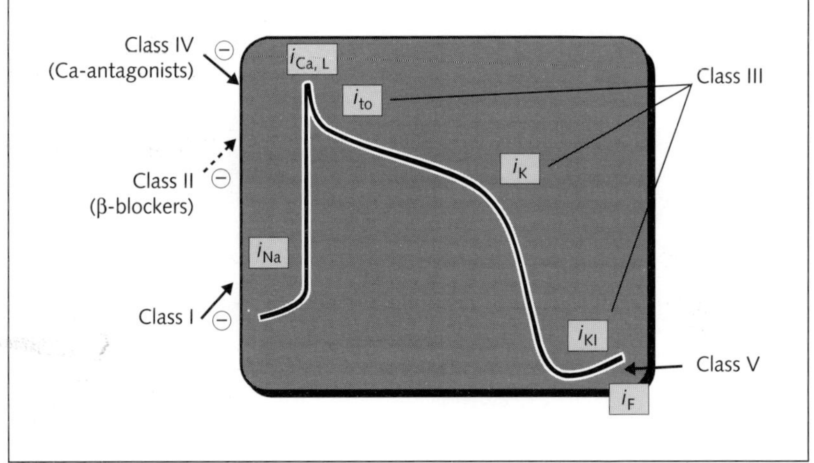

Figure 8.6
Summary of points of action of the various classes of antiarrhythmic drugs (on a Purkinje fibre action potential).

vitro experiments suggest that its effects are due to its action on the Purkinje fibres, serving to reduce their automaticity by its blocking action on the hyperpolarization-activated inward current, i_f. It is not used in human patients.

• Zatebradine. This is a verapamil derivative which induces bradycardia by slowing the rate of diastolic depolarization in the SA node. The basis of this action is inhibition of the hyperpolarization-activated inward current, i_f. This agent has no class III action. It is also not yet used for humans.

Table 8.2 and Fig. 8.6 summarize the points of action of the key antiarrhythmic agents.

8.4 Recent clinical trials of antiarrhythmic agents

The Cardiac Arrhythmia Suppression Trial (CAST) of the late 1980s produced surprising and disconcerting results for the pharmaceutical industry and for cardiologists. It showed that the class I antiarrhythmic drugs encainide and flecainide, when given to those who had already suffered a myocardial infarction caused an increase, instead of the expected decrease, in mortality. These drugs are, however, still used (with caution) in certain clinical conditions in those without coronary artery disease (see Chapter 9).

Subsequent clinical trials have shown that β-blockers lower mortality in both the acute setting of myocardial infarction and in the first year following such an attack. Other recent trials (see above) have, however, indicated that the class III drug *d*-sotalol can lead to increased mortality.

9 | Arrhythmias: clinical considerations

9.1 Introduction

The electrophysiological basis of cardiac arrhythmias was outlined in Chapter 7. Chapter 8 listed and described the antiarrhythmic drugs in common use. This chapter will describe the clinical manifestations of arrhythmias. Unfamiliar terms are defined in the glossary at the end of the book.

9.2 Predisposing factors

There are several factors which predispose an individual to arrhythmia. The key ones are listed below.

9.2.1 Congenital factors

These are present at birth, although not necessarily inherited, and generally require other factors for initiation. Examples include:

• Bypass tracts due to an anatomical abnormality such as those observed in Wolff–Parkinson–White syndrome.
• Inherited cardiomyopathy, an example of which is myotonic dystrophy (an autosomal dominant condition in which there is impaired relaxation of skeletal muscle) which can result in terminal heart failure.

9.2.2 Coronary artery disease

This results in chronic myocardial ischaemia and acute or healed myocardial infarction. The mortality due to ventricular arrhythmia is highest in the first few hours after coronary artery occlusion leading to infarction. A healed myocardium infarction is also a powerful predisposing factor for ventricular arrhythmia if major damage has resulted to the heart. In both cases additional factors are required to initiate ventricular arrhythmia.

9.2.3 Damage to conducting tissue

Fibrosis (usually of unknown origin) or ischaemia may result in damage to the conduction tissue which tends to predispose to bradyarrhythmia.

9.2.4 Long QT syndrome

Hereditary long QT syndrome (Chapter 20) is the best example of a single predisposing factor which can generate an arrhythmia. This autosomal dominant condition is characterized by a resting sinus bradycardia and gross prolongation of the QT interval on the surface ECG. There is a predisposition to the ventricular tachycardia called torsade de pointes (section 9.6.4C). This arrhythmia generally occurs under conditions of low heart rate during which a sudden burst of sympathetic stimulation occurs. In practice this happens when such patients are suddenly awoken from sleep. This type of arrhythmia usually reverts to normal rhythm spontaneously.

9.3 Factors initiating rhythm disturbance

It has been found in subjects undergoing 24-h electrocardiogram (ECG) monitoring that several factors generally interact to produce a rhythm disturbance, although not all of them need to be present. The factors include a slight increase in heart rate due to increased sympathetic drive, low blood potassium (as a consequence of diuretic therapy to prevent heart failure) and ischaemia. The following text provides more specific details.

9.3.1 Sympathetic nervous system activation

If extreme, this can induce arrhythmia even in structurally normal hearts. The mechanism underlying this effect is unclear, although it may be due to an increased calcium 'window' current or activation of a background chloride current which could result in initiation of repetitive early after-depolarizations leading to changes in conduction velocity and refractory periods.

9.3.2 Ventricular premature beat

Following myocardial infarction an excess of premature beats is associated with an increased risk of an arrhythmic death. It has been suggested that if premature beats occur during the vulnerable period (during repolarization) a self-sustaining circus movement can be generated, resulting in ventricular tachycardia. Ventricular ectopic beats can also result in a transient reduction of systemic arterial pressure, giving rise to a reflex increase in adrenergic activity, thereby predisposing to further arrhythmia.

9.4 Maintenance of cardiac arrhythmia

Several factors, given below, play an important role in maintaining arrhythmia.

9.4.1 Structural factors

Generally an abnormal myocardium is needed to perpetuate

ventricular tachycardia. A critical mass of atrial tissue is required to sustain atrial fibrillation. In dogs there is a correlation between the size of the dog and the duration of experimentally induced atrial fibrillations. In humans an increase in atrial size is associated with an increased ability to sustain atrial fibrillation. In horses atrial fibrillation is particularly common and up to a quarter of the shire horses of East Anglia are in atrial fibrillation.

9.4.2 The autonomic nervous system

The autonomic nervous system is also important in perpetuating arrhythmia. If atrial fibrillation or re-entrant supraventricular tachyarrhythmias develop, the sympathetic nervous system is usually reflexly activated because of the drop in blood pressure. Unless the rhythm disturbance ends quickly, a high sympathetic tone becomes established and the arrhythmia is likely to continue.

9.5 The pathological consequences of an arrhythmia

Different subjects can experience an identical arrhythmia but with a very different clinical outcome. This is largely due to differences in cardiac anatomy. A normal subject who experiences atrial fibrillation would be unlikely to experience more than palpitations. If the subject however has moderate or severe impairment of left ventricular function, or severe left ventricular hypertrophy (as a consequence of long-standing hypertension, or hypertrophic cardiac myopathy), it is likely that in addition to experiencing palpitations he or she may also develop heart failure. This is because in the damaged heart up to 40% of left ventricular filling comes from atrial systole in contrast to 10 or 15% in the normal heart. Thus, in damaged hearts atrial fibrillation can lead to a reduction of 30–40% in cardiac output. Taken together with the increase in heart rate, a further reduction in cardiac output results in pulmonary oedema or, if there is coexistent coronary disease, myocardial ischaemia. This sets the scene for more lethal arrhythmias such as ventricular fibrillation.

9.6 Specific arrhythmias

Some types of arrhythmia were briefly introduced in Chapter 7. Table 9.1 gives an outline classification of arrhythmias and the following section puts them in their clinical context.

9.6.1 Extrasystoles (ectopic beats)

Atrial and ventricular extrasystoles are very common. They are found on almost all 24 hour ECG recordings from normal people. They probably have little pathological significance in the normal heart except when very frequent and/or in people with ischaemic heart disease. In diseased hearts ventricular extrasystoles are associated with a higher mortality but there is no evidence that in this situation decreasing ectopic frequency using drugs reduces mortality. Ventricular ectopics are recognized on the ECG by the appearance of a beat with a broad QRS occurring earlier than the next anticipated sinus beat. This is succeeded by a compensatory pause, when the sinus beat falls in the refractory period of the extra beat. The next sinus beat occurs after the pause in its anticipated place but because of the extra ventricular filling that has occurred during the pause, there is a larger than normal contraction, of which the patient is aware. Patients often complain of missed beats rather than extra beats.

Table 9.1
Classification of arrhythmias.

Extrasystoles
Atrial
Junctional
Ventricular
Tachyarrhythmias
Supraventricular
Atrial
Atrial tachycardia
Atrial flutter
Atrial fibrillation
Re-entry (accessory pathway-mediated) tachyarrhythmias
AV nodal re-entry
Wolff–Parkinson–White (AV bypass tract)
Ventricular
Ventricular tachycardia
Ventricular fibrillation
Bradyarrhythmias
Sinus bradycardia
AV block
Intermittent
Partial
Complete

AV, Atrioventricular.

Treatment

Usually none is indicated. Beta-blockers can be used (Chapter 8) though they are not recommended for normal hearts.

9.6.2 Supraventricular tachyarrhythmias

Atrial tachycardia

In 50% of cases this is due to drug toxicity (particularly digoxin overdose); in the remainder it is usually associated with structural heart disease. Occasionally atrial tachycardias can persist undetected for many months and the fast heart rate induces left ventricular dilatation and diminishes left ventricular systolic performance. If normal sinus rhythm is permanently restored, left ventricular function may return to normal. The ECG of an individual suffering from atrial tachycardia is shown in Fig. 9.1b. Figure 9.1a gives normal

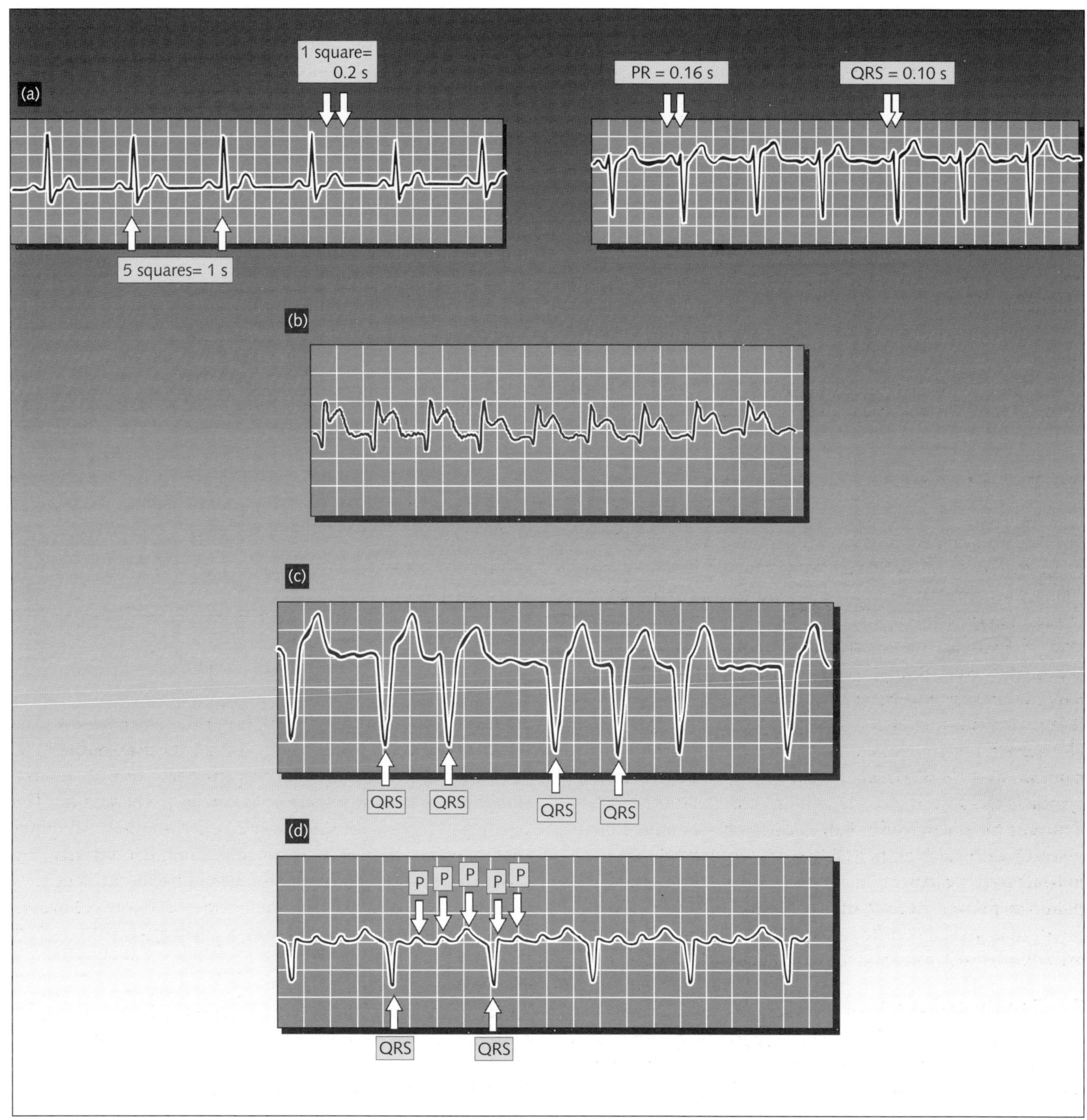

Figure 9.1
(a) Two normal electrocardiogram traces showing the time-scale at which recordings are made and the usual time relations of the P–T waves. (b) Atrial tachycardia is recognized by a P-wave morphology quite different from that in sinus rhythm and usually a shorter P–R interval. (c) Atrial fibrillation is recognized by a totally disorganized baseline and by a very irregular QRS rate. (d) Atrial flutter is characterized by a regular rapid rate of approximately 300/min. A degree of atrioventricular block always occurs such that only every second, third or, as shown here, every fourth beat is conducted to the ventricles. ((a) Redrawn with permission from Hampton, J.R. *The ECG Made Easy*. Churchill Livingstone, Edinburgh.)

ECG recordings for comparison, including the normal time relationships of the various waves.

Treatment

Drugs to slow the ventricular response, e.g. β-blockers, verapamil or digoxin, are given. Restoration of sinus rhythm is attempted, for example, by cardioversion (see below).

Atrial fibrillation

This is probably the commonest sustained arrhythmia (see Fig. 9.1c and d for typical ECGs). Symptoms range from none at all, through irregular palpitations to heart failure. Atrial fibrillation is a potent cause of intracardiac left atrial thrombosis. The thrombi may leave the left atrium to produce systemic emboli, which may, for example, produce a stroke. The mechanism of atrial fibrillation has been described in Chapter 7. A critical mass of atrial tissue is required before re-entry can be sustained (see section 9.4.1 above).

Several approaches exist for the treatment of atrial fibrillation.

• Increase of the conduction block at the atrioventricular (AV) node. Since many of the symptoms arise from a fast ventricular response to the atrial fibrillation, the aim of this is to slow the ventricular response and minimize symptoms. The commonly used drug is digoxin (Chapter 8). Although digoxin has a relatively narrow therapeutic range, it can be safely used in patients with severely compromised left ventricular functions. Alternatively, a β-blocker or a calcium channel blocker such as verapamil or diltiazem can be given.

• Restoration of sinus rhythm. This can be attempted pharmacologically with class I drugs (sodium channel blockers; Chapter 8) that alter conduction properties of the atrium, e.g. flecainide (though its long-term use in patients with coronary artery disease and a previous myocardial infarction is contraindicated), disopyramide or the class III drugs amiodarone or sotalol. The most effective method of restoring sinus rhythm, providing the atrial fibrillation has not been present long and cardiac function is not too severely impaired, is by direct current synchronized cardioversion. This process involves applying a brief electric shock (50–200 J) across the chest in synchrony with the QRS complex to depolarize simultaneously as much atrial tissue as possible (i.e. all that is not in the absolute refractory period). Once atrial repolarization has taken place, firing of the sinus node triggers synchronous atrial depolarization.

• Maintenance of sinus rhythm. Class I antiarrhythmic agents such as quinidine and flecainide and class III agents such as amiodarone can be used with some success (but see the provisos in Chapter 8) to maintain sinus rhythm in those prone to atrial fibrillation.

• Reduction of the incidence of systemic embolism. This is usually done with the vitamin K antagonist warfarin: aspirin can be used but is less effective. A period of anticoagulation should precede attempted cardioversion to minimize the risk of thromboemboli from left atrial thrombi.

• Experimental surgical approaches to atrial fibrillation. Two operations are being developed. The first is known as the corridor procedure and consists of isolating a strip of atrial tissue connecting the sinoatrial node to the AV node. Although the atria continue to fibrillate, the sinus node is intact and the ventricular response to physiological stimuli is normal, so that antiarrhythmic therapy is no longer indicated, although the risk of systemic embolism remains high. The second operation, also still experimental, is known as the maze procedure. Here the atria are divided into strips of tissue too small to sustain re-entrant arrhythmias. The aim is to restore normal sinus rhythm and normal atrial function.

Chronic atrial fibrillation

If atrial fibrillation persists, digoxin is given to reduce AV conduction and hence ventricular rate (see Chapter 8) and anticoagulants to reduce the risk of thrombi.

Atrial flutter

This shows on the ECG as a sawtooth baseline of continuous atrial activity (Fig. 9.1e). In flutter, the atria usually beat at 300 beats/min and the beating is regular (Chapter 7). The refractory period of the AV node usually means that only 150 beats/min are transmitted to the ventricle. The causes and symptoms are much like those for atrial fibrillation but less severe and there is less risk of systemic emboli. Atrial flutter sometimes converts back to sinus rhythm spontaneously.

Treatment is similar to that for atrial fibrillation.

9.6.3 Re-entry (accessory pathway-mediated) tachyarrhythmias

AV nodal re-entrant tachycardia

This occurs when a small (slowly conducting) AV nodal bypass tract allows a circus movement to develop within, or around, the AV node, which sends extra impulses to the ventricle. A typical ECG is shown in Fig. 9.2a.

Termination of this arrhythmia is brought about by enhancing AV conduction blocks. Vagotonic manoeuvres can be tried by the patient and these include the Valsalva manoeuvre (breathing out against the closed glottis), or activation of the diving reflex (plunging the face in cold water). Adenosine (see Chapter 8) is now the treatment of choice to increase AV block as it is so short acting and does not worsen heart failure. Other drugs used to increase AV conduction block include calcium channel blockers (such as verapamil), sotalol, flecainide and disopyramide. Definitive

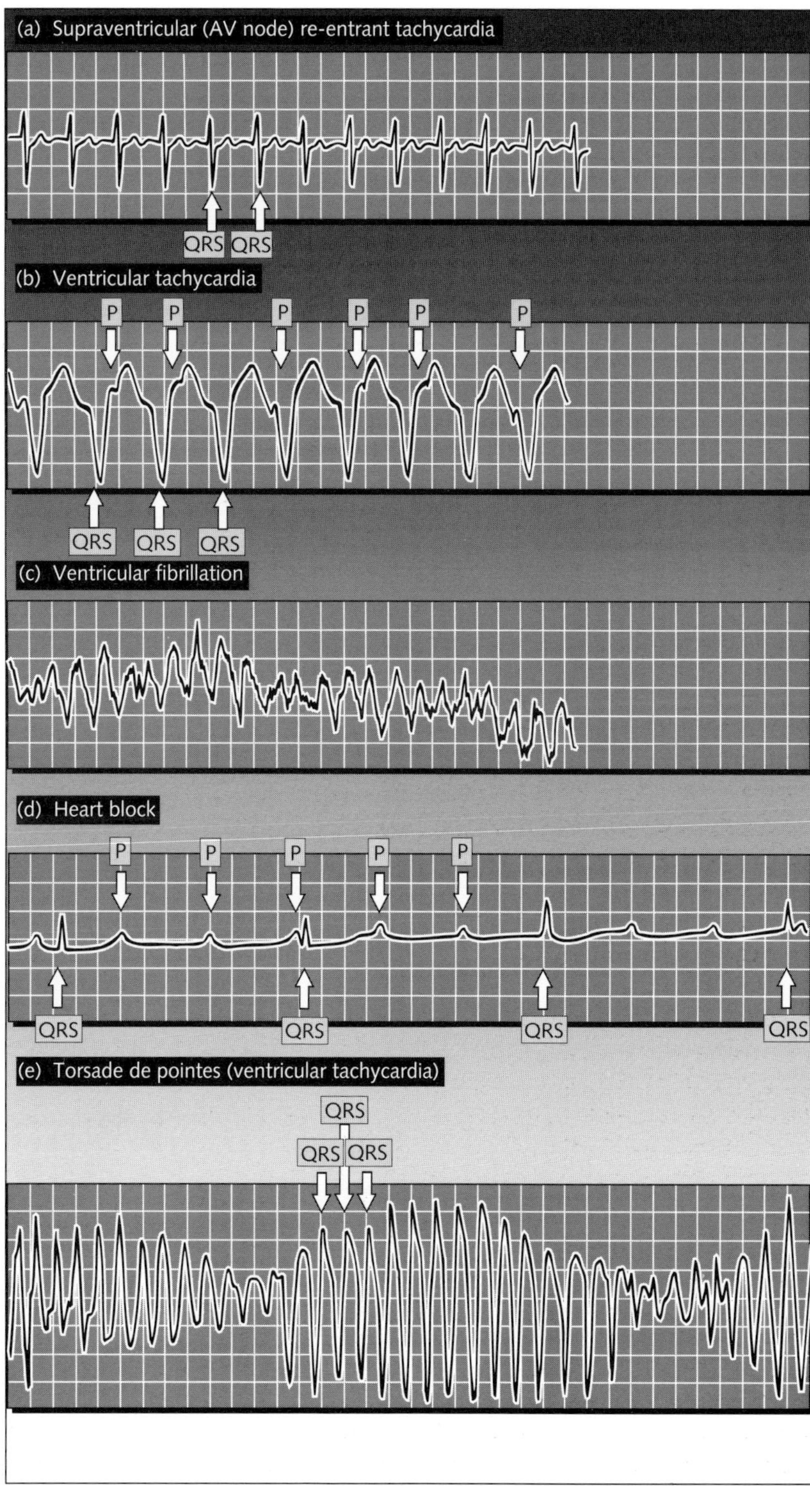

Figure 9.2
(a) Supraventricular arrhythmias, such as the atrioventricular nodal re-entrant tachycardia shown here, are characterized by a regular rapid QRS complex without clear preceding P waves (and thus not sinus rhythm). (b) Ventricular tachycardia is characterized by a broad QRS complex with atrial activity (P waves) occurring independently of this. (c) In ventricular fibrillation there is totally chaotic QRS activity. (d) In complete heart block the atria beat faster than the ventricles and there is no constant relationship between the P waves and the QRS complex. (e) Torsade de pointes.

treatment is now possible using radiofrequency catheters which can be passed through the right femoral vein to the AV node where the slow pathway can be identified and destroyed.

Wolff–Parkinson–White syndrome

This is the second common form of re-entrant tachyarrhythmia. There is a congenital accessory conduction pathway separate from the AV node between the atria and the ventricle. This pathway may be attached to either the left or the right ventricle or to the septum.

Termination of the arrhythmia is often spontaneous. If not, drugs to increase AV block may be used, as above. Definitive treatment is ablation of the accessory pathway using intra-cardiac endocardial radiofrequency catheters (see above).

9.6.4 Ventricular tachyarrhythmias

These are relatively common and may result in serious consequences, including sudden death. Electrocardiographically they are defined as a run of three or more ventricular beats at a rate of more than 120 beats/min. Ventricular tachycardia rarely occurs in the structurally normal heart, if it does it may be relatively benign. This kind of arrhythmia is often diagnosed by giving an intravenous bolus of adenosine which will open an extra potassium channel in the AV nodal cells which will slow or stop conduction of the impulse at this level and so induce transient complete heart block. This either breaks or reveals the nature of most supraventricular arrhythmias but has no effect on ventricular tachycardia. An alternative method of diagnosis is to sense the atria (using an intra-cardiac electrode) and to determine the association between atrial and ventricular activation.

Non-sustained ventricular tachycardia

In this condition there are short self-terminating paroxysms of ventricular tachycardia, usually a manifestation of left ventricular damage, commonly from myocardial infarction or sustained hypertension. They are usually asymptomatic but occasionally patients may experience palpitations, feel faint or occasionally black out.

Sustained monomorphic ventricular tachycardia

This is most commonly found in patients who have had a myocardial infarction and may occur many years after the infarction. Patients experience palpitations, a feeling of faintness or even syncope (fainting). These symptoms often indicate that the cardiac output is inadequate, which can lead to cerebral and myocardial ischaemia. The ventricular tachycardia will then frequently degenerate into lethal ventricular fibrillation. A typical ECG is given in Fig. 9.2b.

For sustained ventricular tachycardia, treatment is in part determined by the state of the patient. If the patient is unwell and in a state of haemodynamic collapse, cardiopulmonary resuscitation should be carried out until direct current cardioversion can be undertaken (which should be done as soon as possible; Fig. 9.3 shows defibrillation successfully

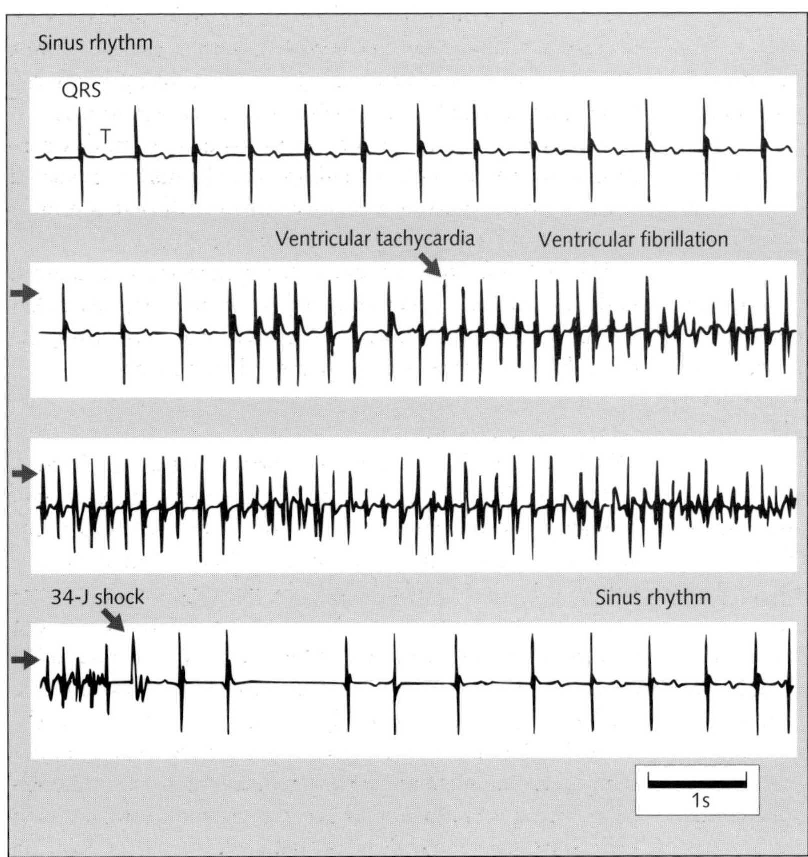

Figure 9.3
Intra-cardiac electrocardiogram of a patient with an implantable cardioverter-defibrillator (ICD) who developed ventricular tachycardia during a visit to the doctor. The ICD delivered a high-energy direct current shock and restored sinus rhythm. (From Roelke, M. & O'Nunain, S.S. (1995) *New England Journal of Medicine*, **332**; 860, with permission.)

converting ventricular tachycardia back to normal sinus rhythm.) For patients who are less unwell, direct current cardioversion still remains a strong option but other possibilities include ventricular overdrive pacing or drug intervention. While such drugs as lignocaine or other class I (Chapter 8) agents or class III (Chapter 8) agents such as amiodarone or sotalol may break the ventricular tachycardia, all of them are negatively inotropic and if they do not stop the ventricular tachycardia, this may result in further deterioration of the patient. Furthermore, they carry a risk of proarrhythmic side-effects. Once ventricular tachycardia has been terminated, the factors underlying it should be treated appropriately by, for example, coronary surgery or postinfarction scar removal.

If drug therapy fails, an implantable cardioverter defibrillator (ICD) can be inserted. This device, through electrodes situated within the right ventricle and superior vena cava, senses the cardiac rhythm. It detects the onset of ventricular tachycardia and responds by pacing the ventricle, thereby overriding the abnormal rhythm. If this fails, the ICD gives an internal direct current shock, of up to 32 J in energy, which usually restores cardiac rhythm. Figure 9.3 shows the ECG from a patient recorded during an incidence of ventricular tachycardia which triggered his ICD so that his sinus rhythm was restored.

Torsade de pointes

This is another form of ventricular tachycardia in which the appearance of the QRS interval is continually changing — hence the name, 'twisting of the points' (Fig. 9.2e). This is commonly seen as a proarrhythmic side-effect of antiarrhythmics such as sotalol or amiodarone (see section 7.6.2). but it also occurs in the setting of the hereditary long QT syndrome (Chapter 20).

Treatment involves either withdrawal of the provoking drug and/or pacing to prevent the precipitating bradycardia or, in the hereditary long QT syndrome, treatment with a β-adrenergic blocker. If this is unsuccessful, left stellate ganglionectomy (to reduce adrenergic input) may be effective.

Ventricular fibrillation

Ventricular fibrillation is characterized by completely disordered and chaotic ventricular activity (associated with an equally chaotic ECG; Fig. 9.2c) and causes total loss of cardiac output. The patient is pulseless and unconscious and appears dead. This can be the end-result of another rhythm disturbance, such as atrial fibrillation with a very high ventricular response in Wolff–Parkinson–White syndrome or sustained ventricular tachycardia in the setting of coronary artery disease, or can occur as a primary event. In 90% of cases, ventricular fibrillation is preceded by tachycardia; in 10% of cases bradycardia precedes it.

Coronary artery disease is the commonest cause of ventricular fibrillation as a complication of acute myocardial infarction. It appears that at least 20% of people resuscitated from an out-of-hospital cardiac event are in ventricular fibrillation by the time the ambulance reaches them. (For a discussion of the underlying causes of ventricular fibrillation, see Chapter 7).

Treatment must be immediate to be successful. If a cardiac defibrillator is available, immediate cardioversion should be attempted. In the absence of a defibrillator, cardiopulmonary resuscitation should be started immediately and continued until sinus rhythm returns or until defibrillation can be attempted. The earlier defibrillation occurs, the more likely it is to be successful and the better the long-term prognosis of the patient. It must then be established whether ischaemia is present and whether the patient requires further treatment, e.g. coronary artery bypass surgery. As with ventricular tachycardia, if drugs prove unsuccessful, or the patient remains at high risk, an automatic defibrillator may be implanted.

9.6.5 Bradyarrhythmias

Sinus bradycardia

The ECG shows normal PQRST with a heart rate of less than 60 beats/min. The commonest cause is physical fitness, and it is not uncommon to see college or university athletes with resting heart rates in the low 40s. Other causes include hypothyroidism and certain drugs (for example, β-blockers). It may, however, also occur when the sinoatrial node is diseased, as for example in sick sinus syndrome. In this syndrome, which may be due to idiopathic fibrosis or associated with coronary artery disease, there are periods of inappropriate bradycardia and inappropriate tachycardia.

The only effective treatment for symptomatic sinoatrial node disease is implantation of a permanent pacemaker which, if there is no associated conducting tissue disease, can be of the type that senses and paces only the atria.

Atrioventricular block

AV block can be intermittent, partial or sustained (complete); see Chapter 7. Symptoms result from the transient, though often profound, loss of cardiac output. Thus at the start of complete AV block there is often a period of time before a slow ventricular escape rhythm originating from the Purkinje fibres intervenes. If the escape rhythm is slow, cardiac output may continue to be inadequate for a period of time, but usually the ventricular escape rate picks up and cardiac output is fairly quickly returned to acceptable levels. Thus the characteristic symptom with intermittent complete heart block or sustained complete heart block is of a complete but transient loss of consciousness of sudden onset and brief duration — the Stokes–Adams attack. The ECG in patients prone to AV block may demonstrate prolongation of the PR interval. In complete heart block the atria beat independently of the ventricles and there is no association between the two, with the atrial rate often being substantially higher than the ventricular rate.

An ECG from a patient with heart block is shown in Fig. 9.2d and other ECGs showing partial and complete heart block were given in Fig. 7.1.

Treatment usually involves insertion of a permanent pacemaker. If there is organized atrial activity it may be appropriate to implant a dual-chamber pacemaker in which the atria can be paced and sensed and the ventricle paced and sensed. Thus, if the patient retains normal sinoatrial node function, the atria will beat normally and this will be sensed by the atrial wire. The ventricle will then be ordered to pace after an appropriate AV-like delay.

For summaries of the relative efficiency and associated adverse effects of the key antiarrhythmic agents referred to in this chapter, see Tables 8.1 and 8.2.

10 Excitation–contraction coupling and mechanoelectrical feedback

10.1 Excitation–contraction coupling

10.1.1 The role of Ca^{2+} ions

It is now more than a century since Ringer showed that the isolated perfused frog heart will not continue to beat unless the perfusion fluid contains 1–2 mmol/l of calcium ions. An extension of his experiment is the quite simple class demonstration that when Ca^{2+} is omitted from the perfusion fluid, the electrocardiogram (ECG) of an isolated frog heart continues almost unaltered, but the contractions cease (Fig. 10.1): the link between excitation and contraction is missing.

It is well-established that in all types of muscle, Ca^{2+} ions are the immediate trigger to contraction. In cardiac, as in skeletal muscle, the binding of Ca^{2+} to troponin loosens the attachment of actin to tropomyosin, thus allowing the actin to interact with the myosin heads and the filaments to move past each other. Details of the present state of knowledge of sliding filament theory are best sought in a text on muscle, but Fig. 10.2 summarizes some key points.

The source of the bulk of the calcium which activates contraction in cardiac muscle is the Ca^{2+} store in the sarcoplasmic reticulum (SR) and it is released shortly after the surface membrane is depolarized. The free Ca^{2+} concentration within the muscle rises from the resting level of about 100 nmol/l (10^{-8} mol/l) to well above 1 mmol/l (10^{-6} mol/l), the level at which the myofilaments are activated.

Details of the link between surface membrane depolarization and the release of the SR store of Ca^{2+} are becoming clearer. In cardiac muscle, though not in skeletal muscle, the entry of Ca^{2+} ions from the external fluid is an essential part of that link.

10.1.2 The intracellular membranous system of cardiac muscle

Invaginations of the surface membrane, T-tubules, perforate the interior of cardiac muscle cells. They are about 250 nm wide, 5–10 times wider than those of skeletal muscle, and are located at the level of the Z lines not, as in skeletal muscle, at

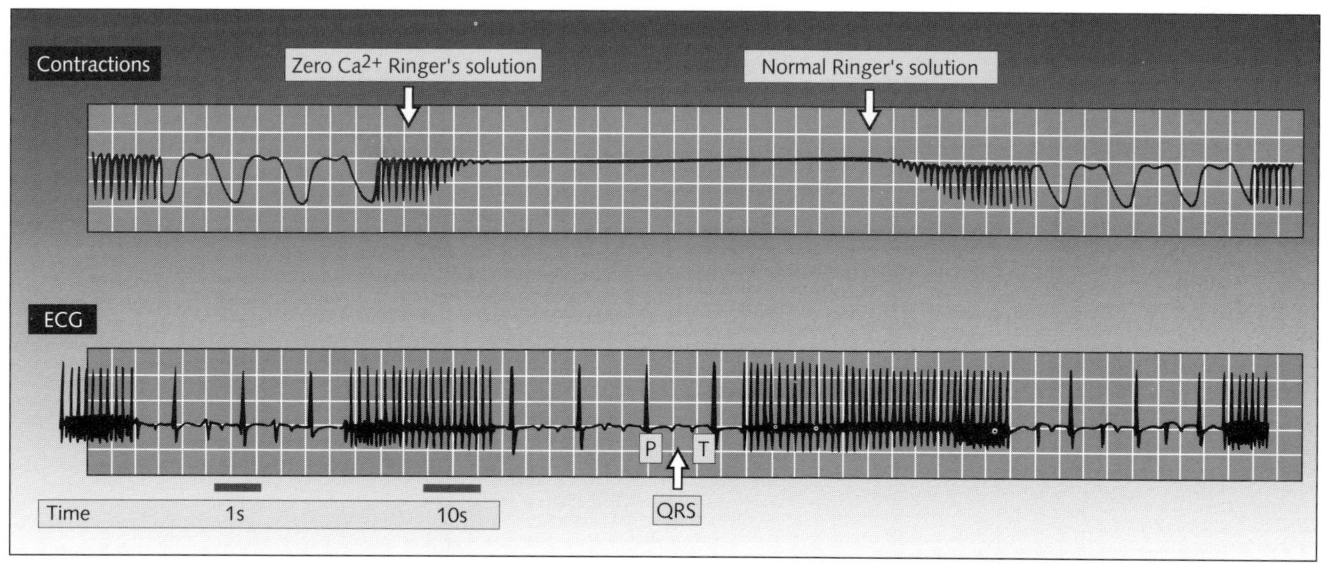

Figure 10.1
Records from a spontaneously beating isolated frog heart perfused with Ringer's solution through a cannula tied into the sinus venosus. (Above) Movement recorded from a hook inserted into the ventricle, attached to an electromechanical transducer (contraction down the page). (Below) Electrocardiogram recorded from the surface of the heart. Ringer's solution with the calcium omitted was introduced at the arrow. The electrocardiogram continued but the contractions ceased.

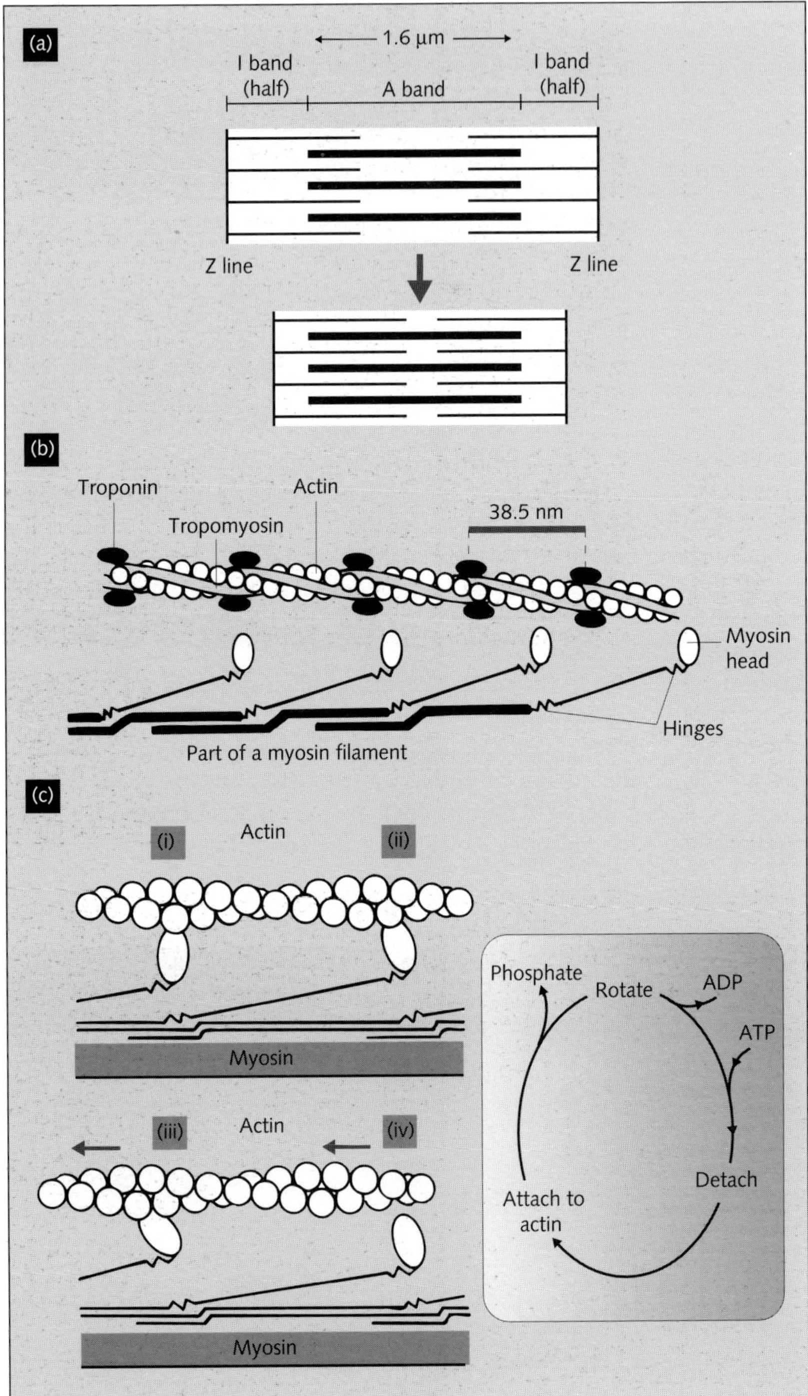

Figure 10.2
Interaction of actin and myosin filaments to cause contraction. (a) The diagram shows the thick and thin filaments of a sarcomere sliding between one another. The thick filaments (A band) are made of the protein myosin and the thin filaments (I band), principally of actin. (b) Each thin filament is composed of a double helix of F actin, a polymer of globular G actin, together with two further proteins, tropomyosin and troponin. The thick filament is made up of the rod-like parts of myosin molecules. Flexibly attached myosin heads project from the thick filament at regular intervals. When Ca^{2+} concentration rises, the Ca^{2+} ions bind to troponin and this displaces the tropomyosin, exposing active sites on the actin filaments. The myosin heads bind to these sites forming cross bridges, ATP is split and the two sets of filaments slide between one another. (c) How sliding is thought to occur. The myosin head, which acts as an ATPase, splits ATP to ADP and phosphate and stores energy. It attaches to an active site on an actin filament (i) and uses the stored energy to swivel on its flexible attachment and so move the actin filament relative to the myosin filament (ii) and (iii). The myosin head then loses ADP, binds more ATP and detaches from the actin filament (iv). The right-hand panel shows cross-bridge activity during contraction. (Redrawn from Keynes, R.D. & Aidley, D.J. (1991) *Nerve and Muscle*, 2nd edition. Cambridge University Press, Cambridge.)

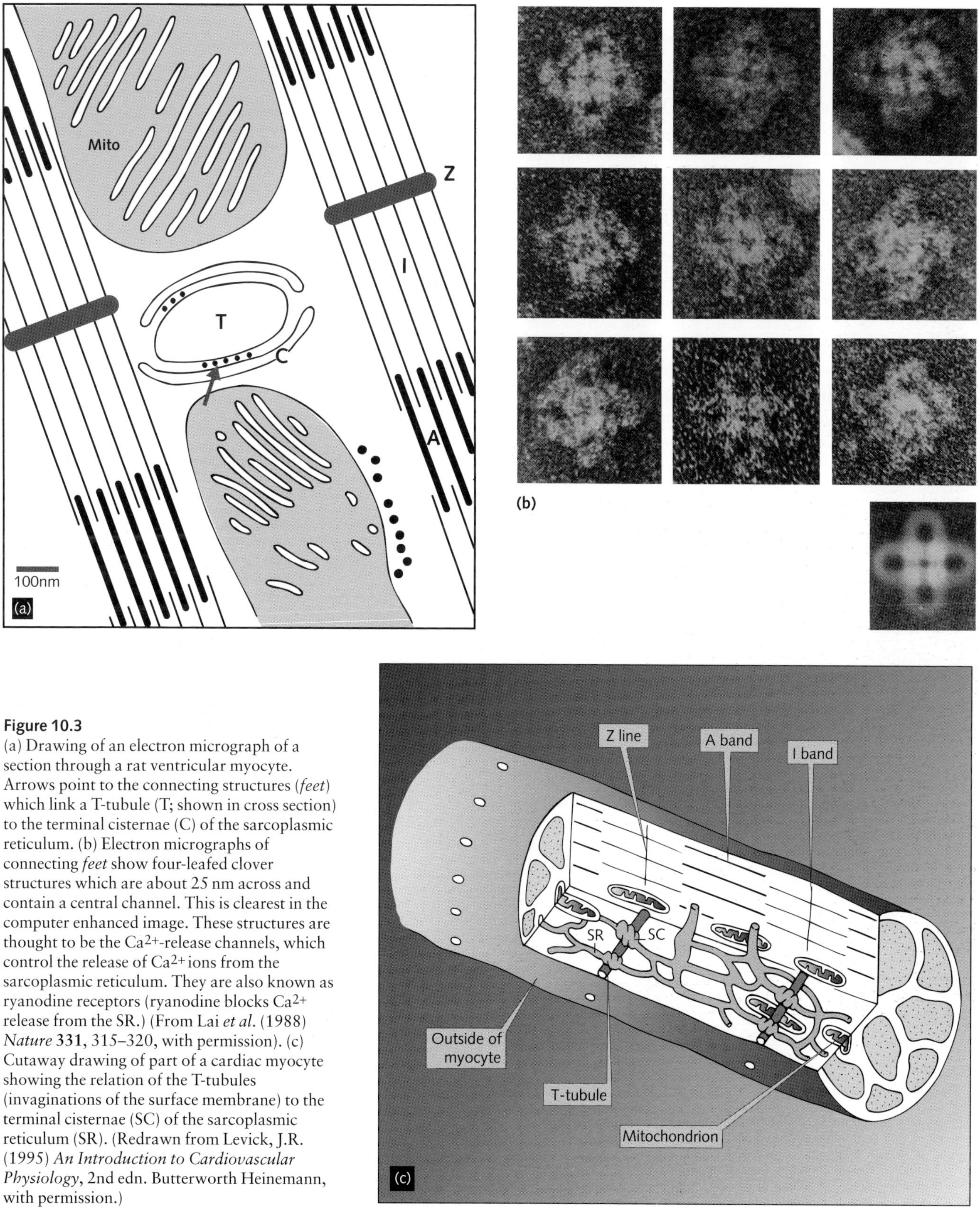

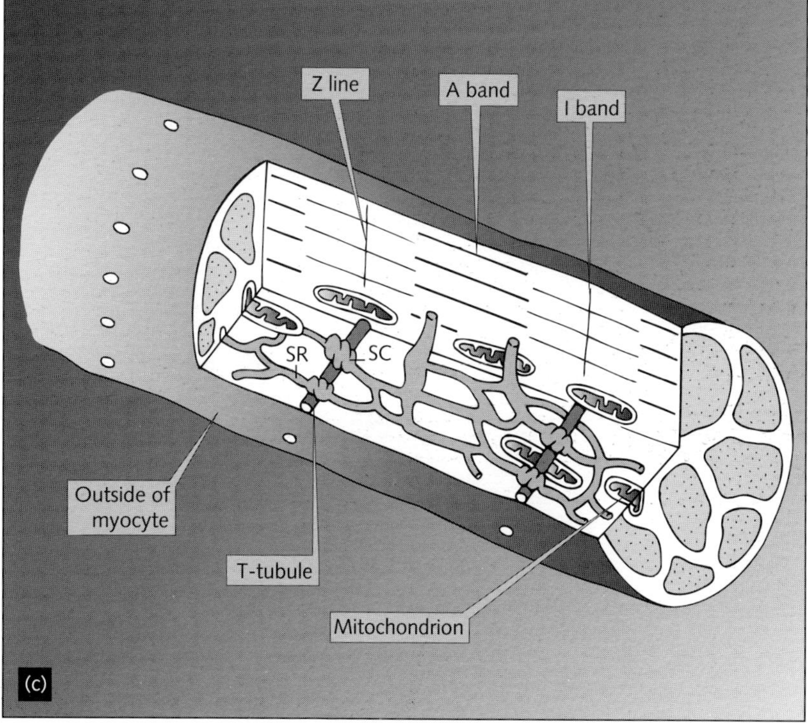

Figure 10.3
(a) Drawing of an electron micrograph of a section through a rat ventricular myocyte. Arrows point to the connecting structures (*feet*) which link a T-tubule (T; shown in cross section) to the terminal cisternae (C) of the sarcoplasmic reticulum. (b) Electron micrographs of connecting *feet* show four-leafed clover structures which are about 25 nm across and contain a central channel. This is clearest in the computer enhanced image. These structures are thought to be the Ca^{2+}-release channels, which control the release of Ca^{2+} ions from the sarcoplasmic reticulum. They are also known as ryanodine receptors (ryanodine blocks Ca^{2+} release from the SR.) (From Lai *et al.* (1988) *Nature* **331**, 315–320, with permission). (c) Cutaway drawing of part of a cardiac myocyte showing the relation of the T-tubules (invaginations of the surface membrane) to the terminal cisternae (SC) of the sarcoplasmic reticulum (SR). (Redrawn from Levick, J.R. (1995) *An Introduction to Cardiovascular Physiology*, 2nd edn. Butterworth Heinemann, with permission.)

the junctions of the A and I bands. A T-tubule (near the Z line) is well shown in the electron micrograph in Fig. 3.3a. The T-tubules come into close contact with sacs of SR called terminal cisternae and electron-dense 'feet' (or junctional channel complexes) can be seen to span the gap between the two sets of membranes (Fig. 10.3a,b). The terminal cisternae (which in skeletal muscle have been shown to contain stores of Ca^{2+}) form part of the extensive closed network of SR tubules which surround the myofilaments (Figs 10.3 and 10.4).

10.1.3 The bridge between T-tubule membrane and sarcoplasmic reticulum

Using 'skinned' cardiac cells, from which the surface membrane has been removed with detergent, it has been shown that increase in ionized calcium concentration causes release of further Ca^{2+} from the stores in the SR (calcium-induced calcium release). The Ca^{2+}-release channel in the SR membrane is blocked by low concentrations of the alkaloid, ryanodine. The molecules to which ryanodine binds have been isolated and examined under the electron microscope. They resemble four-leaved clover, each with a central pore (Fig. 10.3b). They appear to be identical in size and shape to the 'feet' spanning the gap between T-tubule and SR terminal cisternae membranes.

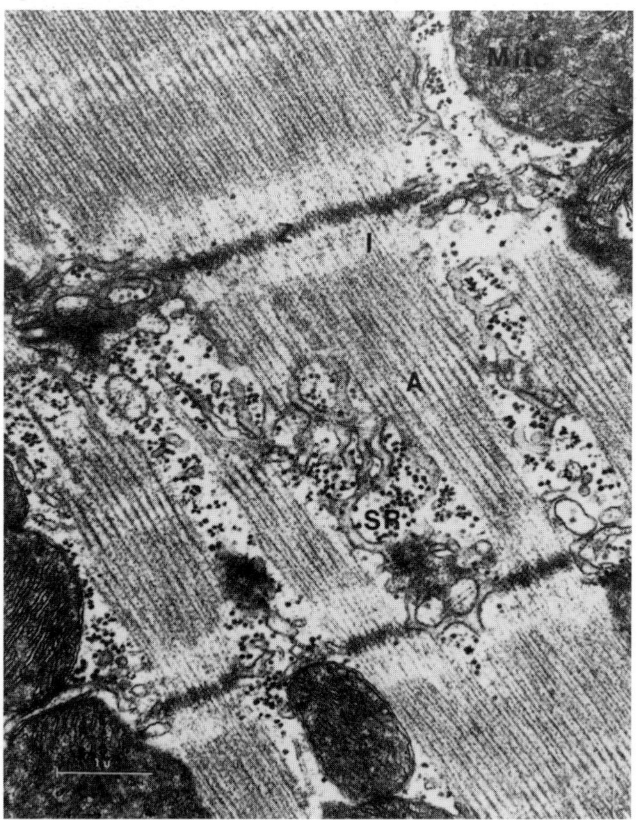

Figure 10.4
Sarcoplasmic reticulum (SR) (electron micrograph). Scale bar 1 μm. (From Katz, A.M. (1977) *Physiology of the Heart*. Raven Press, New York.)

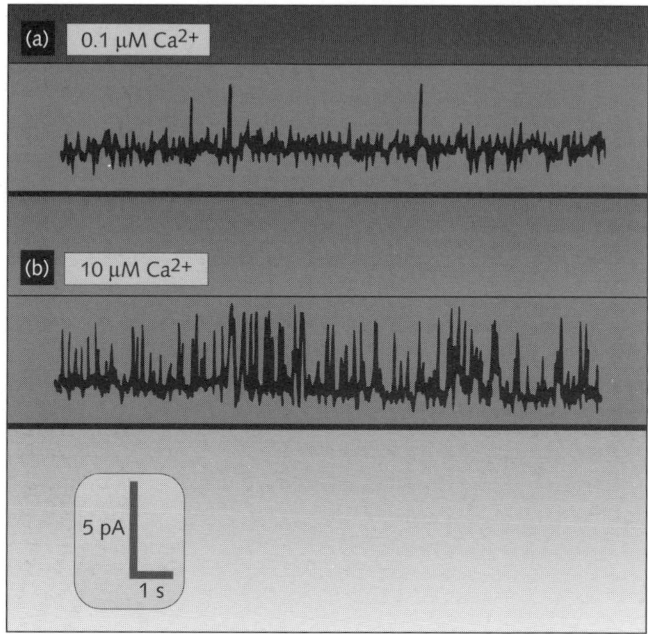

Figure 10.5
Record of the opening of a single Ca^{2+}-release channel which had been extracted from the sarcoplasmic reticulum membrane of cardiac muscle cells and inserted into a lipid membrane. Increasing the concentration of Ca^{2+} on the cytosolic side of the channel causes a great increase in the frequency with which the channels open. (Courtesy of Dr R. Sitsepesan.)

10.1.4 Sequence of events in excitation–contraction coupling

The sequence of events is thought to be as follows: depolarization of surface membrane and hence of the T-tubule membrane opens voltage-sensitive Ca^{2+} channels so that calcium ions enter the cardiac cell. This leads to a conformational change in the 'feet' (Ca^{2+}-release molecules) such that Ca^{2+} very rapidly floods out of the SR to activate the contractile mechanism. This process can now be studied using fluorescent dyes and confocal microscopy to visualize 'calcium sparks'. (See p. 121 Eisner & Trafford (1996).)

After the contraction phase, the free calcium concentration is returned to resting level, bringing about relaxation, Ca^{2+} ions are pumped back into the longitudinal tubules of the SR by a Ca^{2+}-adenosine triphosphatase (ATPase) pump and then moved along to the terminal cisternae again, ready to be released by the next wave of depolarization. Some Ca^{2+} ions are removed by exchange for external Na^{+} across the surface membrane and some also by a Ca^{2+}-ATPase pump in the surface membrane of the muscle cell.

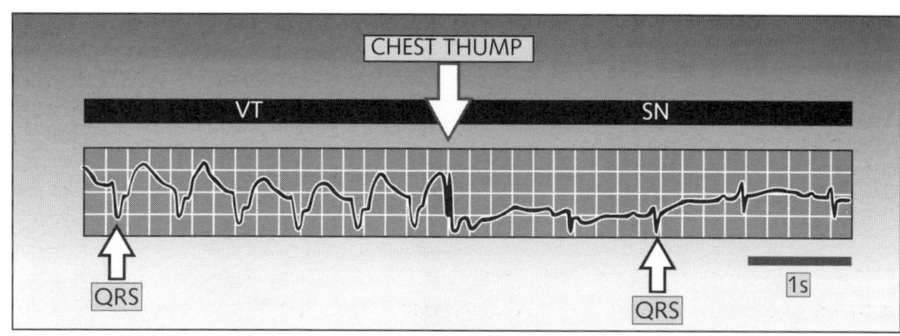

Figure 10.6
Restoration of normal sinus rhythm (SN) in a patient in ventricular tachycardia (VT) by mechanical stimulation of the heart (a thump on the chest). (From Pennington *et al.* (1970) *New England Journal of Medicine* **283**; 1192–1195, with permission.)

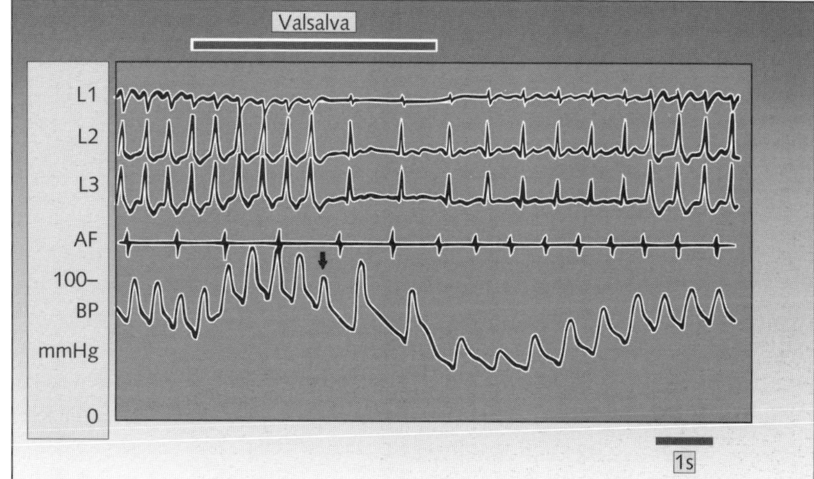

Figure 10.7
Temporary termination of ventricular tachycardia by the Valsalva manoeuvre (expiration against a closed glottis). L1 to L3, electrocardiogram recordings from the body surface; AF, natural atrial frequency of the heart; BP, arterial blood pressure. (From Waxman, M.B. *et al.* (1980) *Circulation* **62**; 843–851, with permission.)

10.1.5 The calcium-release channel in the sarcoplasmic reticulum membrane

This can be isolated and inserted into an artificial membrane (a lipid bilayer). Here, the openings and closures of the channel can be recorded: openings are more frequent when the calcium concentration rises and in the presence of such compounds as caffeine (Fig. 10.5).

10.2 Mechanoelectric feedback

10.2.1 Mechanical activation of cardiac cells

In 1915, Francis Bainbridge showed that injection of fluid into the jugular veins of anaesthetized dogs led to a temporary increase in heart rate. He concluded that an increase in venous return caused a reflex acceleration of heart rate 'caused by impulses arising within the heart'. This came to be known as the Bainbridge reflex but it was later found that in isolated hearts also, stretch of the sinoatrial node region gives rate acceleration so the effect is not—or not only—a reflex but a more direct response of cardiac cells to stretch.

An impressive example of a mechanical stimulus causing electrical excitation of cardiac cells is shown in Fig. 10.6, where a thump on the chest reverted ventricular tachycardia to normal heart rhythm. It appears that the transient stretch-induced depolarization of all non-refractory cells reset the rhythm as would depolarization from a defibrillator. In emergencies, quiescent hearts can be repeatedly activated by chest compressions and the process can be continued for a considerable time.

Stretch-induced excitation can also be proarrhythmic, as illustrated in Fig. 10.7, which shows a patient with ventricular tachycardia who performed the Valsalva manoeuvre (expiration against a closed glottis), a procedure which increases intrathoracic pressure and reduces ventricular filling. The reduction in wall tension allowed the heart to revert to its normal rhythm for a few beats, after which the initial level of ventricular filling was re-established, stretching the myocardium again and triggering the tachycardia.

10.2.2 Stretch-activated channels

Ion-channel activity in response to various different types of stretch has been demonstrated in the membranes of a variety of different types of cardiac cell. Either the membrane within

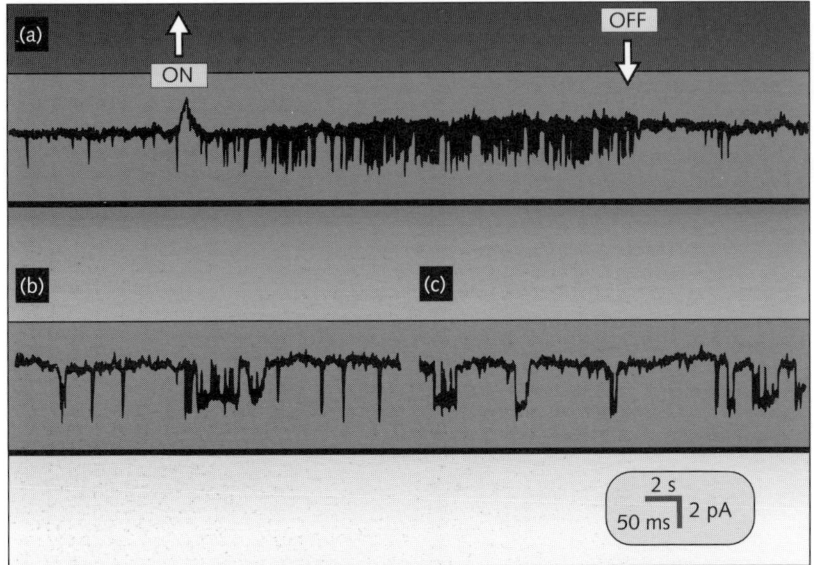

Figure 10.8
Activation of a stretch-activated non-selective cation channel in a neonatal rat ventricular myocyte by applying negative pressure to the inside of the recording pipette to stretch the membrane within the pipette's orifice. (From Craelius, W. *et al.* (1988) *Bioscience Reports* 8; 407–414, with permission.)

a patch pipette aperture can be stretched by applying negative pressure to the pipette, or cell volume can be increased, usually by placing the cell in a hypo-osmotic solution so that it swells, or the whole cell can be longitudinally stretched by attaching its ends to carbon fibres or microglass tools.

Figure 10.8 shows some of the first records of stretch-activated channel activity in mammalian cardiac cells. The channels were in the membrane of neonatal rat ventricular myocytes and negative pressure applied to the patch pipette opened channels which were found to pass cations non-selectively. This would be expected to produce a depolarization of the membrane potential. Indeed, mechanical activation of these channels has been shown to trigger action potentials in isolated cardiomyocytes. Direct stretch of the membrane patch or longitudinal stretch of the whole cell activates channels which usually seem to be of this type (cation conducting) while many volume-activated channels which open in response to osmotically induced swelling or to injection of fluid into the cell are selective for chloride ions. This could be, at any rate partially, a volume-control response, since loss of chloride will be followed by loss of Na^+ ions and water, and it has been found that block of these volume-activated chloride channels facilitates further increase in cell volume. Opening of Cl^- channels will, however, also cause a depolarization (as in the case of the catecholamine-activated chloride current mentioned in Chapter 12) and it is interesting that chloride channels have been shown to be activated in isolated sinoatrial cells of the rabbit on inflation through the patch pipette.

10.2.3 The possible importance of fibroblasts

There is some evidence that fibroblasts within heart tissue could be involved in sensing stretch. Fibroblasts are especially numerous in the pacemaker region and also in scar tissue, and they can be shown to be both mechanically sensitive and linked to myocytes by electrically conducting nexi. They may sense stretch and depolarize the myocytes to which they are connected.

The functional importance of these and other findings awaits further investigation and requires more selective blockers of stretch-activated channels than are currently available. Network computer simulations using the system shown in Fig. 20.1 suggest that activation of a limited number of stretch-activated channels could provoke ectopic firing and be a cause of arrhythmia.

11 Functional aspects of cardiac muscle contraction

11.1 Introduction

The mechanical events in the cardiac cycle were described in Chapter 2; functional aspects of cardiac muscle contraction will now be considered.

Table 11.1 lists values of cardiac output and heart rate at rest and in maximum exercise. Notice that in exercise heart rate increases proportionally more than does stroke volume and that the maximum heart rate and the end-systolic volume (ESV) are the same for athletes as for non-athletes.

11.2 Graphical representation of cardiac muscle function

There are various ways of representing cardiac muscle function graphically, most of which bear a relationship to the length–tension curves of cardiac muscle which are outlined in Fig. 11.1a. These curves can be replotted for the whole heart as pressure–volume curves and within them the pressures at the different points in the cardiac cycle can be filled in. This has been done for both right and left ventricles in Fig. 11.1b. Once round the loop in an anticlockwise direction represents one heart beat. The area of such a loop (pressure × volume) is proportional to the external work done by the ventricle. This is much less for the right than for the left ventricle, since the pressures in the pulmonary circulation are much lower than

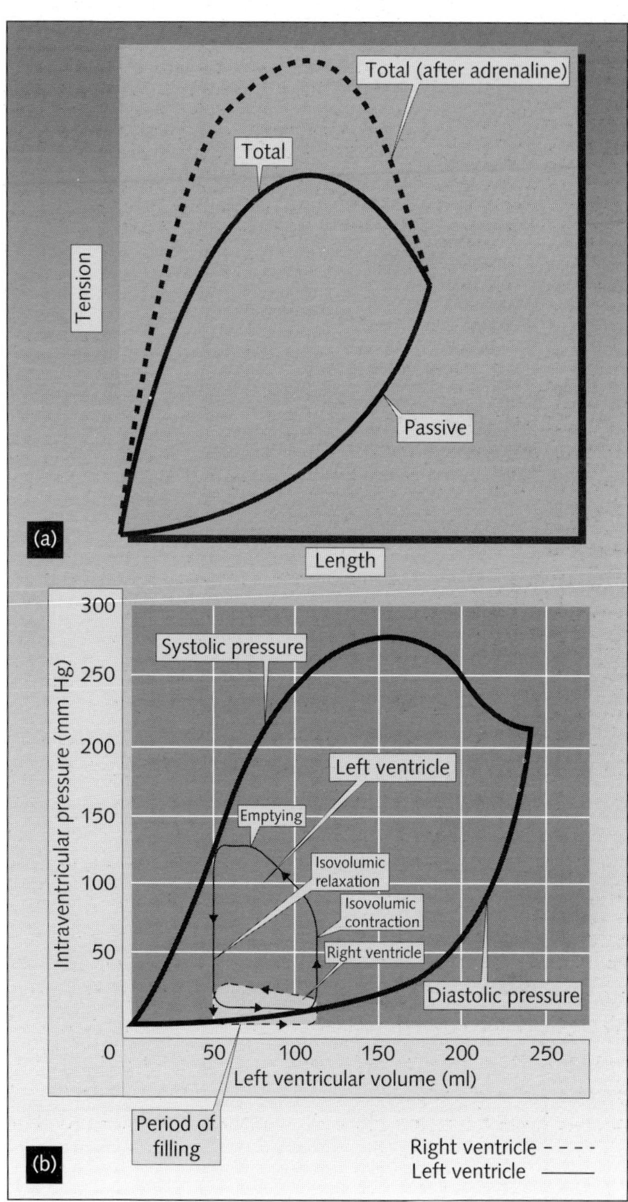

Figure 11.1
(a) Length–tension curves for cardiac muscle (total and passive). (b) Normal pressure–volume curves for right and left ventricles placed within curves for the maximum systolic and diastolic pressures (left ventricle) which can be generated isometrically at different end diastolic volumes. Note that the maximum pressure curves are very similar to the length–tension curves in (a).

Table 11.1
Cardiac output, heart rate, stroke volume, end-diastolic volume (EDV) and end-systolic volume (ESV) at rest and in exercise for non-athletes and for trained athletes. (From Bray, J.J. *et al.* (1994) *Lecture Notes on Human Physiology*, 3rd edn. Blackwell Scientific Publications, Oxford.)

	Cardiac output (l/min)	Heart rate (beats/min)	Stroke volume (ml)	EDV (ml)	ESV (ml)
Non-athlete					
Rest	5	70	70	130	60
Maximum exercise	22	180	120	140	20
Trained athlete					
Rest	5	40	120	200	80
Maximum exercise	36	180	200	220	20

in the systemic, though, of course, the volume of blood moved is the same for each ventricle.

11.3 Frank–Starling mechanism—heterometric regulation

Otto Frank (1895) and later E.H. Starling (1914) investigated length–tension relationships using frog myocardium and isolated perfused mammalian heart, respectively. Their basic finding (known as Starling's law of the heart or, better, the Frank–Starling effect) was that the more cardiac muscle is stretched, the more tension it produces. Their observations showed that heart muscle normally works on the rising phase of the length–tension curve (Fig. 11.1a), unlike skeletal muscle where the resting length is usually at the peak of the length–tension curve.

In an isolated perfused heart, the preload (venous pressure or atrial pressure) can be altered and the outflow against a constant afterload (representing arterial pressure) measured. Although Starling did not himself consider mechanical work, the mechanism he described in such experiments is best shown as a plot of stroke work against mean atrial pressure (which itself determines the degree of stretch of the ventricular muscle at the end of diastole). Such a curve (Fig. 11.2) is a form of length–tension curve; it is called a Starling curve. Both this curve and the pressure–volume curves are types of ventricular function curves. Figure 11.3 shows the effect on the left ventricular pressure–volume curve of increasing end-diastolic volume: more external work is now being done by the heart.

This kind of regulation of the strength of the heart beat is sometimes called intrinsic control of stroke volume or heterometric autoregulation (because it occurs from different initial lengths of the muscle). It is a very important self-regulatory feature of heart contraction. It ensures that:

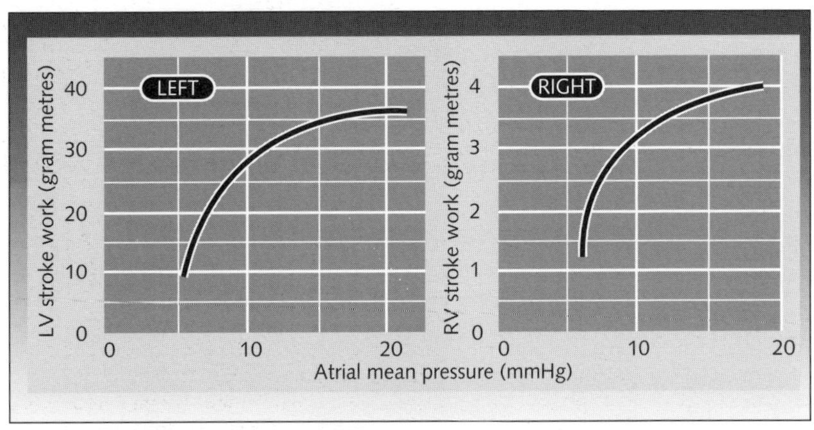

Figure 11.2
Starling curves (stroke work versus atrial pressure) for left and right ventricle. Atrial pressure determines the degree of stretch of the ventricular muscle at the end of diastole.

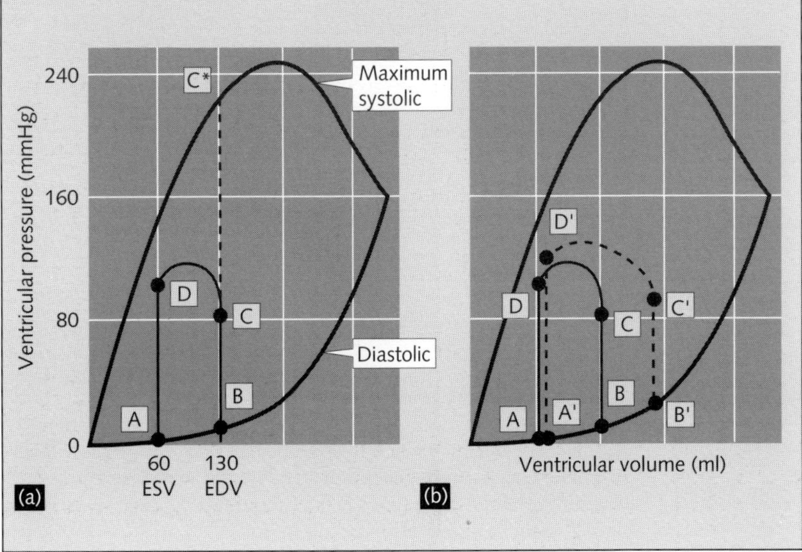

Figure 11.3
Left ventricular volume–pressure curves. (a) ABCD indicates the normal cardiac cycle. ESV, end systolic volume; EDV, end diastolic volume. C* is the ventricular systolic pressure achieved by an isometric contraction if the aortic valve remains closed. (b) Change in normal volume–pressure curve for left venticle (solid line) when end diastolic volume is increased from B to B′.

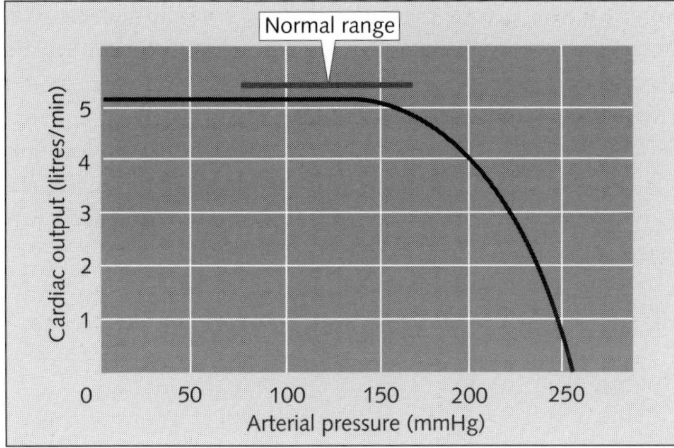

Figure 11.4
The output of the heart is independent of changes in arterial pressure over the normal daily range of 80–170 mmHg. This is because the most important factor determining the amount of blood pumped by the heart is atrial pressure (which determines the amount the ventricle is stretched; Frank–Starling effect).

1 The output of the heart keeps up with the volume of blood delivered to it.
2 Stroke volume is maintained against rises in arterial pressure (Fig. 11.4).
3 The outputs of the two sides of the heart are matched.
4 Any transient changes in interbeat interval (and hence of cardiac filling) are immediately compensated for by a stronger or less forceful beat.
5 Loss of pressure generation resulting from the Laplace relationship (see below) is compensated for.

The way in which ventricular function curves are altered by catecholamine action will be dealt with in Chapter 12.

11.4 Cellular basis for Starling's law

The mechanism by which the force of contraction of heart muscle increases with initial length was once believed to result from changes in myofilament overlap (as does the length–tension relationship of skeletal muscle) but it is now thought that the more important relationship is that between the activation of the contractile proteins by calcium and muscle length. This effect stems from the properties of cardiac troponin C. Thus in 'skinned' cardiac fibres (fibres with the external membrane removed), the affinity of troponin C (see Fig. 10.2 and its legend) for Ca^{2+} has been shown to increase with increasing length and substitution of cardiac muscle troponin C by skeletal muscle troponin C in chemically prepared skinned fibres greatly diminishes the Starling effect (enhanced performance at greater length). In addition to increasing the sensitivity of the myofibrils to Ca^{2+}, greater initial length may also increase Ca^{2+} release from the sarcoplasmic reticulum.

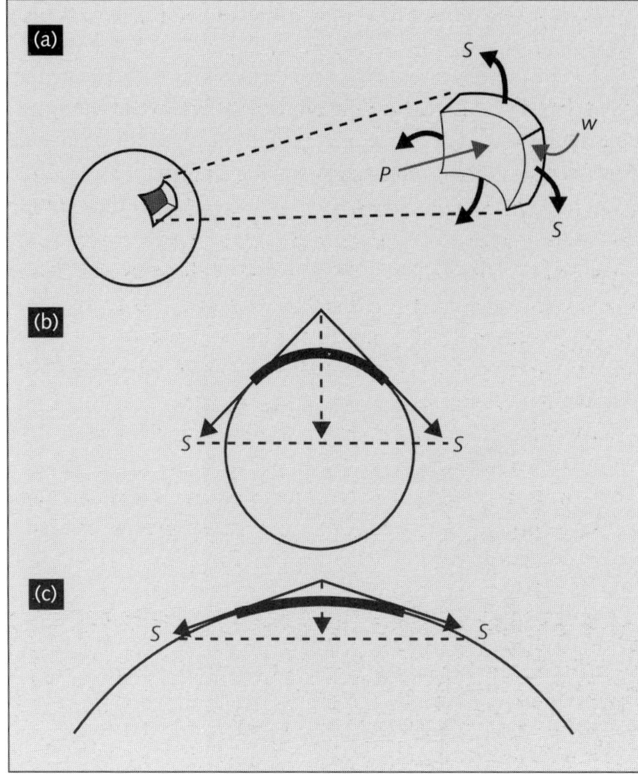

Figure 11.5
Relation between wall tension (or wall stress), *S*; pressure, *P* and curvature of a hollow sphere. (a) illustrates circumferential wall stress in a hollow sphere. (b) shows how the wall tensions (tangential arrows) give a resultant inward stress equal and opposite to pressure within the sphere. (c) Increase of the radius of the sphere reduces curvature and thus reduces the inward component of the wall stress. *w*, wall thickness. (From Levick, J.R. (1995) *An Introduction to Cardiovascular Physiology*, 2nd edn. Butterworth Heinemann, with permission.)

11.5 Law of Laplace and the heart

The law of Laplace, which relates wall tension (wall stress) and internal pressure in all hollow organs, is also applicable to the heart. Laplace's law can be stated:

$$S = \frac{Pr}{2w}$$

The wall tension, *S*, is the force per unit length tangential to the vessel wall and it opposes the distending force, *Pr*, which tends to pull apart a theoretical longitudinal split in the vessel wall. *P* is the transmural pressure (pressure outside the vessel minus pressure inside) and *r* is the radius of the vessel. In the case of the heart, wall thickness, *w*, must be taken into account (Fig. 11.5).

The law of Laplace has some important consequences for the heart:

1 The rise in pressure during the ejection phase of the cardiac cycle (Fig. 11.1b) is due to the physical effect of the change in ventricular size, not to any increase in the strength of muscle contraction. As the radius gets smaller and the wall thicker, extra pressure is generated for the same tension in the ventricular wall.

2 When the heart becomes dilated in disease, the heart muscle must generate increased tension to pump against even normal arterial pressure, which exacerbates the problems already present by creating an extra demand for energy and oxygen.

3 Trained athletes develop hypertrophied hearts, but here the increased wall thickness compensates for the increased radius and no extra tension need be developed to generate a given pressure.

12 The nervous control of heart rate and force

12.1 Introduction

Heart rate and force of contraction can be increased by the sympathetic nerves supplying the heart and decreased by the parasympathetic nerve supply (positive and negative chronotropic and inotropic effects). These nerves form the efferent limbs of various reflexes, particularly those involved in the control of blood pressure. Autonomic effects are also very important in heart disease and in exercise.

Measured plasma concentrations of catecholamines at rest are 1 nmol/l adrenaline and 2–3 nmol/l noradrenaline, rising 10–15-fold during severe exercise. Working heart muscle close to sympathetic nerve endings may well see levels that are considerably higher than these. Meaningful measurements of plasma acetylcholine (ACh) cannot be made since ACh is rapidly and completely broken down by acetylcholinesterases in synaptic regions or else is reabsorbed into nerve endings. Threshold levels of ACh which give detectable effects on membrane currents are around 1 nmol/l.

12.2 Control of heart rate

12.2.1 Sympathetic control of heart rate

Sympathetic fibres to the heart leave the spinal cord at the thoracic level and synapse within the ganglia of the cardiac plexus. The postganglionic fibres innervate the cardiac muscle, releasing catecholamines on stimulation. These act predominantly on β_1-receptors although β_2 and α receptors are also present on the myocytes.

Figure 12.1a shows the effect of catecholamine application on the spontaneous electrical activity of a sinoatrial (SA) node cell. (For details of pacemaking in the SA node, see Chapter 5). Figure 12.1b demonstrates that in SA node cells, catecholamines (β_1-agonists) produce a very large increase in inward calcium current ($i_{Ca,L}$) as they do also in other parts of the heart. This increase in calcium current is partly responsible for the increased rate of firing, by speeding up the last part of the pacemaker depolarization and the (calcium-based) upstroke of the SA node action potential. In atrial, and in particular ventricular, muscle the large increase in force of contraction resulting from this increase in $i_{Ca,L}$ (the positive inotropic response to catecholamines) is very important. It is further considered in section 12.3.1, below.

Catecholamines are also found to increase the hyperpolarization activated inward current, i_f, by shifting its activation curve in a positive direction, so that at a given potential more of this current will be activated and thus contribute to the acceleration of SA node firing. They also increase the time-dependent potassium current, i_K, thus speeding up repolarization. This last effect might be thought to be counterproductive but it is important at high heart rates (catecholamines can produce up to three times the normal rate) for without it the action potentials and hence refractory periods would be prolonged, limiting the firing rate achieved. There is also some evidence that the potassium current, i_K, decays more rapidly under the influence of catecholamines.

12.2.2 Parasympathetic control of heart rate

The heart rate is normally under tonic parasympathetic control. Thus administration of atropine, which blocks the parasympathetic transmitter ACh, raises the heart rate from about 70 to 100 beats/min. Cardiac parasympathetic fibres originate in the medulla oblongata and pass in the vagus nerve to synapse with postganglionic cells within the heart itself, which then act on muscarinic M_2-receptors.

Figure 12.2a shows the slowing of the spontaneous SA nodal activity produced by ACh at a concentration of 50 nmol/l (5×10^{-8} mol/l). At this low concentration (not far above its threshold concentration of 1–3 nmol/l), ACh acts chiefly on two of the membrane currents which contribute to SA nodal pacemaking: it reduces i_f and $i_{Ca,L}$.

At higher ACh concentrations, an additional membrane conductance is activated, giving an 'extra' potassium current, termed $i_{K,ACh}$, which hyperpolarizes the maximum diastolic potential and further slows the pacemaker depolarization. Figure 12.2b shows these effects when 100 nmol/l (10^{-7} mol/l) ACh is applied to an isolated SA nodal cell. Still higher doses of ACh activate sufficient $i_{K,ACh}$ channels to cause profound hyperpolarization with temporary stoppage of SA nodal firing. The pathway for this action of ACh has been much studied and is shown in Fig. 12.3. A G-protein (guanosine triphosphate-binding protein) linked to the ACh receptor which lies near the $i_{K,ACh}$ channel in the cell membrane acts directly upon it to increase the probability of channel opening. There is no cascade of intracellular reactions linking receptor and channel so the action is very rapid.

Whereas the right vagus preferentially innervates the SA node, which is on the right side of the heart, fibres from the

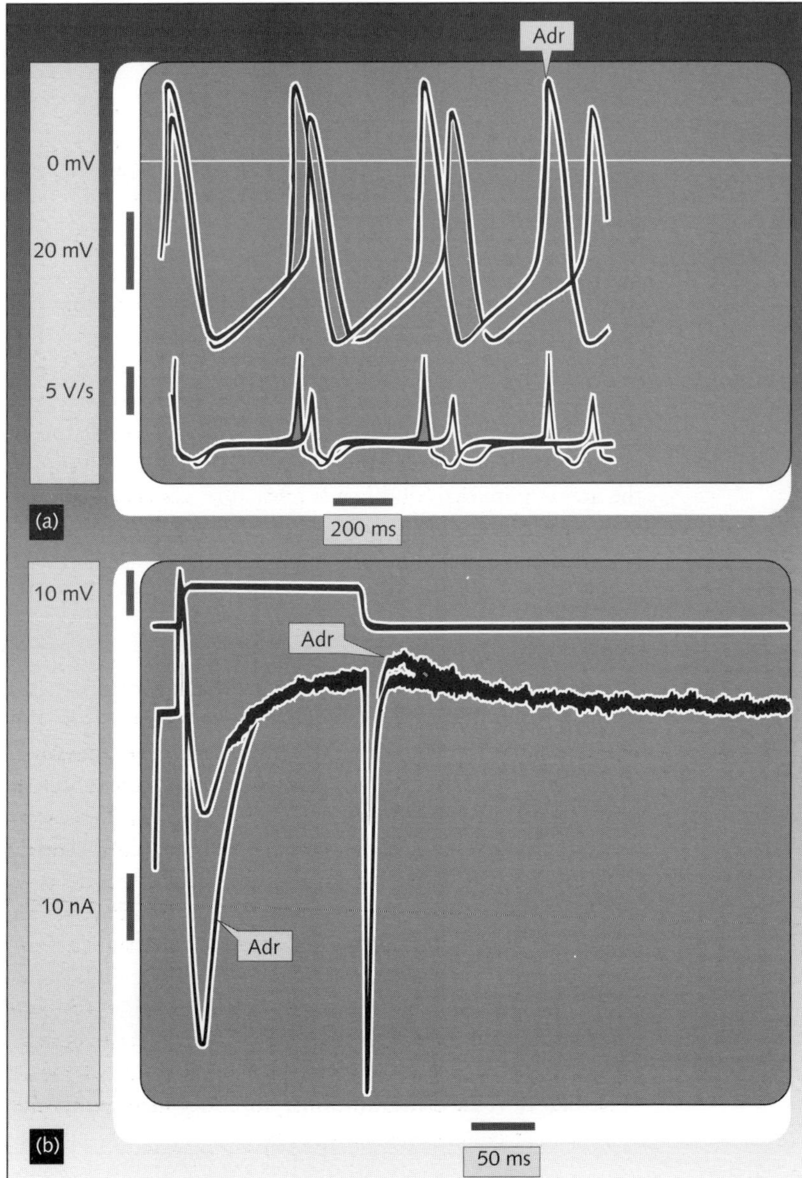

Figure 12.1
(a) *Above*. Spontaneous electrical activity recorded from the sinoatrial node. Two traces are superimposed: a normal trace and (arrowed) after addition of 10^{-7} mol/l adrenaline. *Below*. Rate of change of voltage; the increase in this in adrenaline reflects the large increase in inward calcium current during the upstroke. (b) Voltage clamp of a small SA node preparation. A depolarizing clamp pulse of 10 mV (above) activates inward calcium current, $i_{Ca,L}$, and outward potassium current, i_K (seen clearly as the current 'tail' on return to the holding potential). Two traces have been superimposed, the second after addition of 10^{-7} mol/l adrenaline which increased both $i_{Ca,L}$ and i_K.

left vagus innervate preferentially the AV node. Left vagal stimulation can suppress conduction of impulses through the AV node and lead to complete heart block (Fig. 12.4). The mechanism of ACh action on AV nodal cells is thought to be similar to that on SA nodal cells, with possibly a predominance of reduction of $i_{Ca,L}$, which reduces the conduction velocity of the impulses through the nodal tissue.

12.3 Control of cardiac force

12.3.1 The effect of catecholamines on stroke volume (positive inotropic effect; homeometric regulation)

Catecholamines or sympathetic stimulation cause heart muscle to contract with much greater force. This is sometimes called extrinsic regulation of stroke volume or, because the muscle starts from the same length, homeometric regulation (in contrast with the heterometric regulation discussed in Chapter 11). It results in a shift of the Starling curves (plots of stroke work against left atrial pressure) upwards and to the left, as shown in Fig. 12.5. From a given length, the muscle fibres contract with much greater force—their contractility is increased. Decrease of tonic sympathetic discharge to the ventricle can shift the curve in the opposite direction, reducing ventricular contraction strength by about 20%. Plotted as pressure–volume loops, adrenaline can either increase stroke

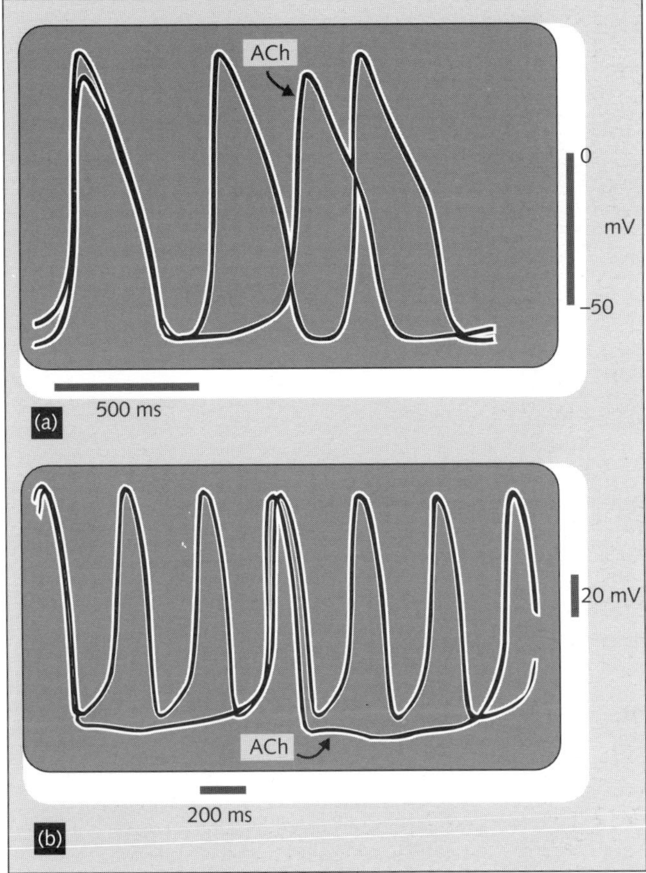

Figure 12.2
(a) Acetylcholine 5×10^{-8} mol/l on spontaneous electrical activity of a sinoatrial node cell. (b) Acetylcholine 10^{-7} mol/l on sinoatrial node cell.

volume (Fig. 12.6a) or maintain a normal stroke volume against an increased arterial pressure (Fig 12.6b). In both cases the area within the loop increases—more work is being done.

The best way of judging cardiac performance is by the initial velocity of shortening of the muscle. Contractility is closely related to the maximum velocity of contraction that can be produced from a given resting length. Velocity of shortening itself is not easy to measure in the whole heart and a more useful way of assessing contractility is to measure the rate of change of pressure as the heart contracts. Left ventricular pressure is plotted against time in Fig. 12.7 for a normal heart, a hypodynamic heart and a heart under the influence of adrenaline. Maximum rate of change of pressure (dP/dt) (slope of the tangent to the steepest portion of the ascending limb of the curve) shows striking differences and is often used to assess contractility.

12.3.2 Cellular basis for the positive inotropic effect

The powerful effects of catecholamines on cardiac muscle are the end-result of a well-documented biochemical cascade of reactions illustrated in Fig. 12.8. This starts within the membrane, when receptor activation, via a G-protein, stimulates the enzyme adenylate cyclase. This raises the level of cyclic adenosine monophosphate (cAMP) within the cell which activates protein kinase to phosphorylate and thus open Ca^{2+} channels in the membrane. The very large increase in L-type calcium current caused by β-adrenergic agonists has already been described in the SA node cell in connection with the acceleration of rate (Fig. 12.1b). Increase in Ca^{2+} current is not confined to the SA node, it occurs in all heart muscle cells when β_1-adrenergic agents are present. When more Ca^{2+} ions enter the cardiac cell, more are released from the SR. The higher the concentration of free calcium rises, the more forcefully the myofilaments will be activated. The Ca^{2+}-ATPase pump that moves calcium ions back into the SR is also boosted by catecholamines.

12.3.3 Parasympathetic negative inotropic effect

Reduction of $i_{Ca,L}$ by parasympathetic stimulation will reduce the strength of contraction (negative inotropic effect). It is well-established that parasympathetic stimulation can reduce sympathetically augmented $i_{Ca,L}$ (by virtue of reduction of shared second messengers in the intracellular cascade, as shown in Fig. 12.8) and hence reduce contraction, but there is controversy as to whether it can reduce basal $i_{Ca,L}$ (i.e. in the absence of prior sympathetic stimulation).

The consensus of opinion is that such reduction of basal calcium current can be seen in the SA node and in the atrium, probably because in such regions intrinsic levels of adenylate cyclase and hence cAMP are high, but only in some species can it be detected in ventricular cells.

12.4 Other autonomic effects on the heart

12.4.1 Catecholamine-induced chloride current

A chloride current induced by catecholamines has been identified in ventricular tissue. E_{Cl} (the reversal potential for chloride ions) lies between –30 and –50 mV in ventricular cells. Negative to E_{Cl}, this channel will contribute an inward and therefore potentially arrhythmogenic current (as Cl^- ions move out of the cell) while at potentials positive to E_{Cl} it will contribute an outward current which will tend to shorten action potential duration. This could counteract the action potential lengthening which results from high levels of catecholamines and consequent calcium loading of the cells and early after-depolarizations (see Chapter 7). ACh decreases this current and so tends to increase action potential duration.

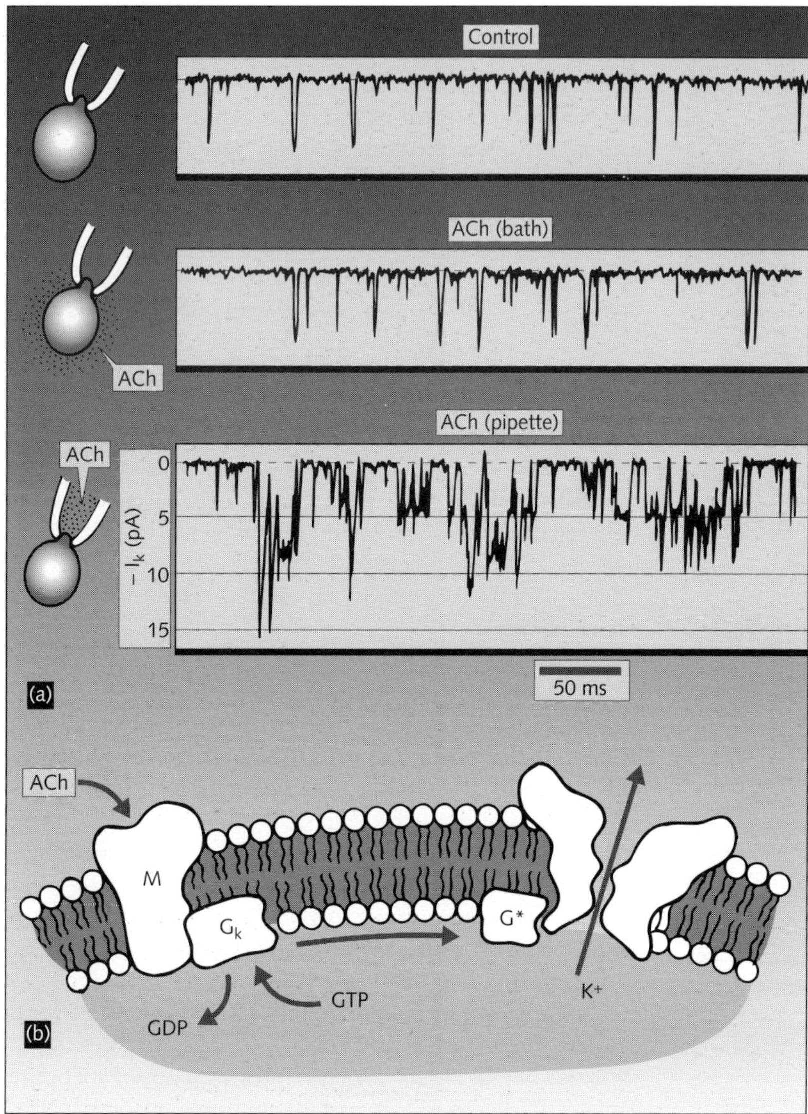

Figure 12.3
(a) Records of single $i_{K,ACh}$ channels in a cell-attached patch on a rabbit atrial cell. Top record: before any acetylcholine is applied; there are occasional channel openings. Middle record: during addition to the fluid perfusing the bath of 100 nM acetylcholine; the frequency of channel opening is unchanged. Bottom record: acetylcholine has been washed out of the bath and the recording pipette perfused with 10 nM acetylcholine; there is a great increase in frequency of channel opening. This shows that the activation of $i_{K,ACh}$ channels occurs very locally. (b) Scheme of the sequence of events in the muscarinic activation of an $i_{K,ACh}$ channel. (Redrawn from Hille, B. (1992) *Ionic Channels of Excitable Membranes*, 2nd edn. Sinauer Associates Inc., Sunderland, MA.)

12.5 Autonomic tone and balance

12.5.1 Autonomic tone

The heart rate is normally restrained by parasympathetic tone and thus cutting the vagal supply causes the rate to rise by 40–50% (from 70 to 100 beats/min).

12.5.2 Autonomic balance

The balance and interaction between sympathetic and parasympathetic outflow to the heart are important. The details of the cellular pathways of parasympathetic and sympathetic action (see, for example, Fig. 12.8) have indicated some of the points (e.g. raising or lowering cAMP) at which interaction between the two systems can occur. There is also evidence for prejunctional interaction: substances released from parasympathetic nerve fibres can interact with receptors on sympathetic nerve terminals to modulate the release of noradrenaline and vice versa.

12.5.3 Autonomic balance in heart disease

There is evidence that autonomic outflow and balance can alter in such conditions as ischaemic heart disease or after myocardial infarction. Acute ischaemia stimulates intracardiac sensory endings leading to reflex augmentation of both parasympathetic and sympathetic outflow to the heart. Since parasympathetic effects predominate in the SA node and sympathetic effects do so in the ventricle, this can give a reduced heart rate (parasympathetic action) coupled with

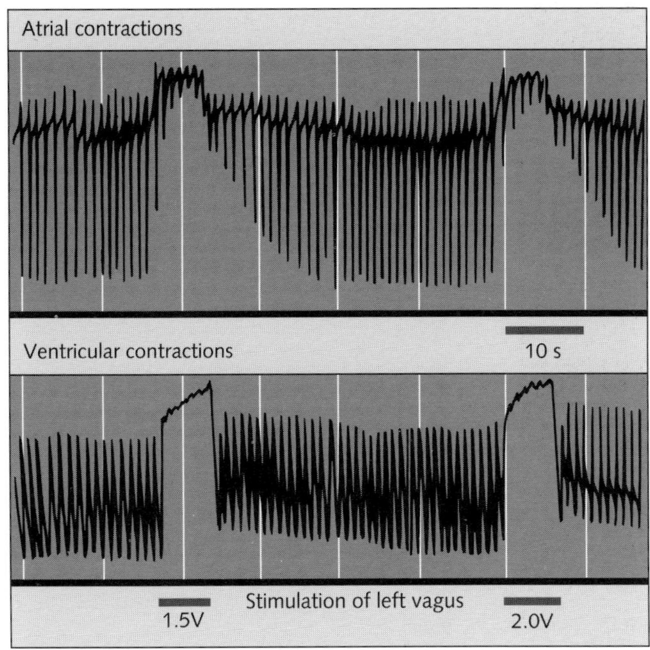

Figure 12.4
Records of the contractions of the right atrium and the ventricle of a terrapin heart (downward movement of trace signifies contraction). When the left vagus is stimulated, the atrium continues beating while the ventricular beats cease for several cycles. Parasympathetic outflow to the atrioventricular junction blocks impulse conduction by the same processes (chiefly reduction of inward calcium current, $i_{Ca,L}$ and activation of $i_{K,ACh}$) that cause the reduction in strength of the atrial contractions during vagal stimulation, with a gradual recovery afterwards.

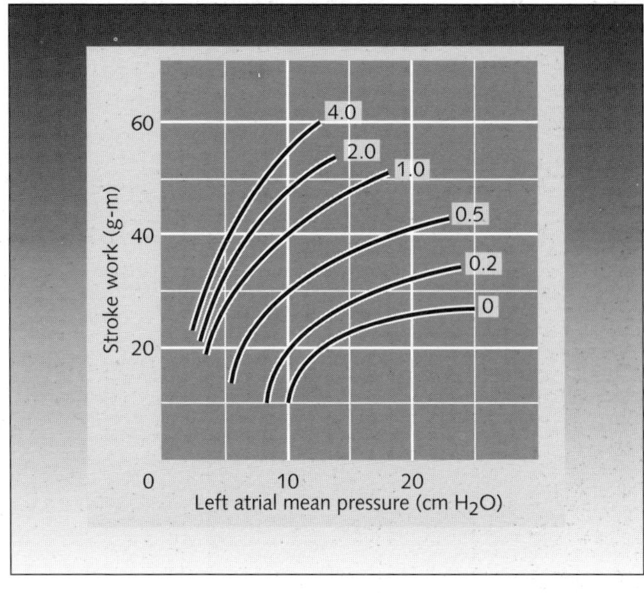

Figure 12.5
When the sympathetic nerves to a dog's heart are stimulated, the Starling curves (stroke work plotted against left atrial pressure, the determinant of end diastolic volume) shift upwards and to the left. Thus at a given venous filling pressure, the heart does more work. Numbers show the frequency of nerve stimulation in Hz. (Redrawn with permission from Sarnoff, S.J. & Mitchell, J.H. (1962) *Handbook of Physiology Cardiovascular System*, vol. I. American Physiology Society, Bethesda, MD.)

shortened ventricular refractory period (sympathetic). Nevertheless, a reflex bradycardia in response to acute ischaemia has been associated with a better prognosis in humans and with a lower incidence of ventricular fibrillation in animal models. One of the possible benefits of parasympathetic activation during acute ischaemia could be reduction of the catecholamine-induced chloride current discussed in section 12.4.1 above.

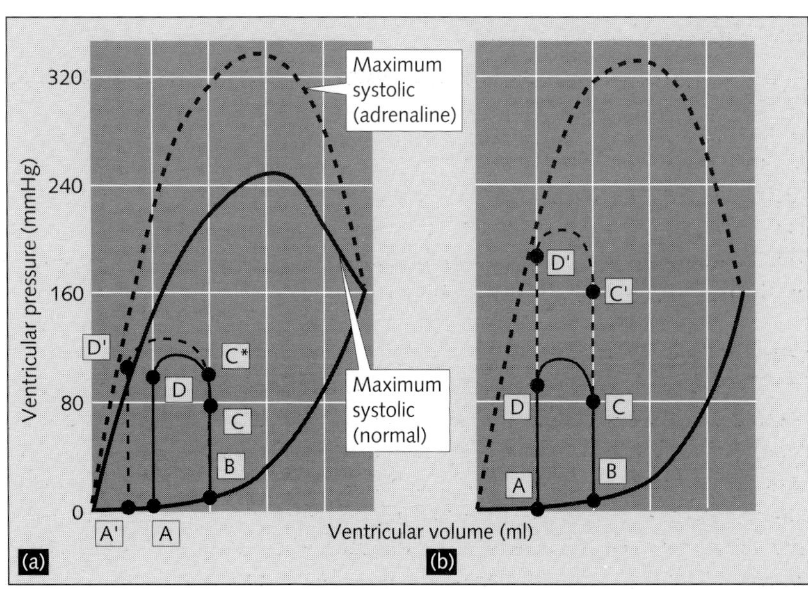

Figure 12.6
Effect of catecholamines on ventricular pressure–volume curves. (a) There is an increased stroke volume with the pressure–volume cycle A′B C′D′A′. (b) A normal stroke volume is maintained in the face of an increased afterload of the magnitude of C′.

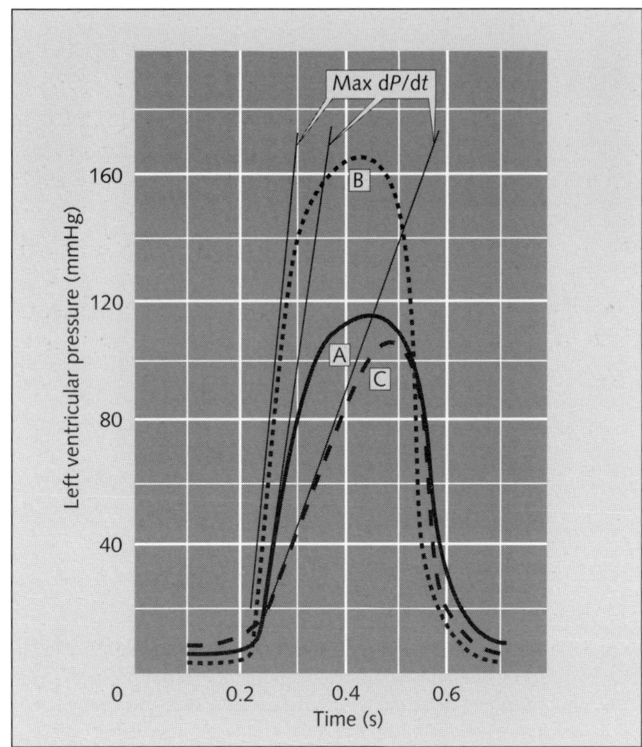

Figure 12.7
Left ventricular pressure curves with tangents drawn to the steepest points on the rising phases to show maximum d*P*/d*t* (rate of change of pressure), A, Normal heart. B, Under sympathetic stimulation. C, Hypodynamic heart (heart failure).

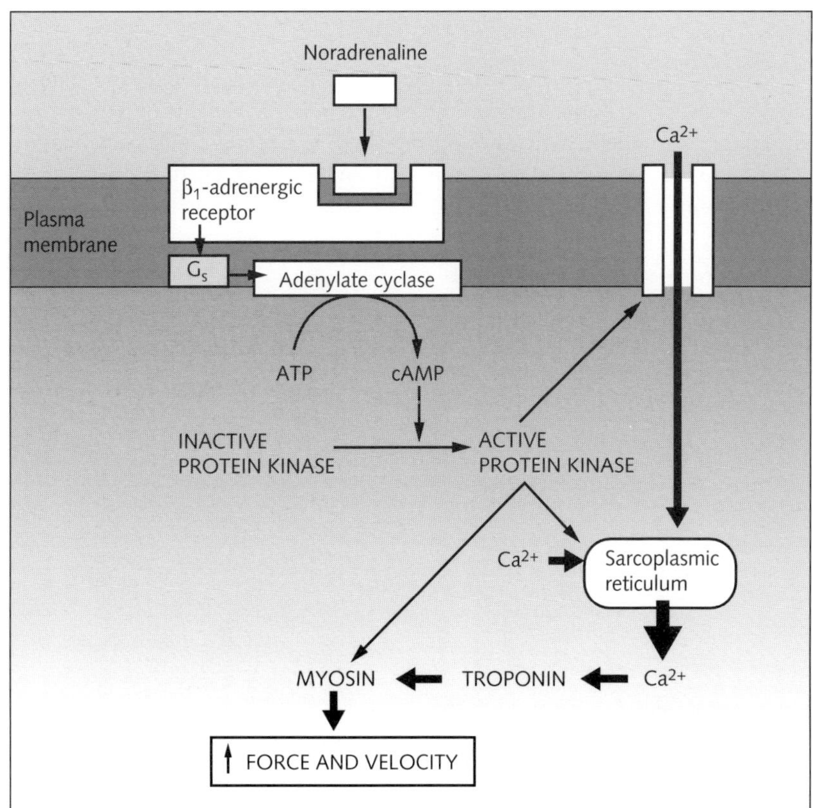

Figure 12.8
'Cascade' of reactions between β-receptor and Ca^{2+} channel.

12.5.4 Autonomic balance in exercise

Heart rate increases greatly during exercise, typically from about 70 beats/min at rest to about 190 beats/min. There is a profound increase in sympathetic outflow to the heart and a withdrawal of parasympathetic tone. Whether the latter is complete during severe exercise is still debated; injections of atropine at peak exercise cause a further increase in heart rate, but there is some evidence that atropine itself can activate calcium current and inhibit $i_{K,ACh}$.

12.5.5 Effects of training on autonomic balance

Trained subjects have lower heart rates for a given severity of exercise (peak rate in severe exercise is approximately 5% lower in a trained than in an untrained subject) and lower heart rates at rest. The mechanism whereby these reductions are achieved remains controversial. It has been suggested that prolonged exposure to higher levels of catecholamines (as will occur during physical training) could lead to a desensitization of β-receptors or to a reduction in their numbers (down-regulation). Alternatively, there may be increased parasympathetic outflow or an actual change in the intrinsic rate of nodal pacemaking after training, possibly related to higher degrees of stretch associated with the larger trained heart.

13 | Measurement of cardiac output

The methods now most commonly used to measure cardiac output are variants of dilution methods, in which a known amount of a substance is introduced into the blood stream and its dilution calculated by measuring its concentration in serial samples at the same sampling point. If the injection is made into a vein and the samples taken from an artery, it is assumed that thorough mixing has occurred during the passage through each side of the heart and through the pulmonary circulation. In this way the amount of blood passing this point can be simply calculated and hence a value for the cardiac output can be reached. The blood flow in litres per minute (F) is given by the formula:

$$\text{Flow} = \frac{\text{Amount injected}}{\text{Mean concentration} \times \text{time for one circulation}}$$

Although dye dilution has been largely replaced clinically by thermodilution methods (see below), the principle is the same and we will first consider a dye dilution experiment.

Venous blood (10 ml) is withdrawn from the basilic vein through a cannula: 5 ml is kept as a blank and to the other 5 ml is added 25 mg of Evans blue, a dye which will not leave the blood system once injected. Blood (1 ml) containing 5 mg dye is injected rapidly into the basilic vein and samples of arterial blood are then taken at intervals of 0.5–2.0 s into a series of tubes. These are centrifuged, together with the blank sample, and the dye concentration determined photocolorimetrically. The concentrations are plotted on semilogarithmic paper, as shown in the solid curve in Fig. 13.1. The dotted curve gives the dye concentration in another experiment in which the subject performed work. Each curve reaches a peak (the one in the work experiment does this more quickly), declines and then starts to rise again as blood containing the dye starts to recirculate. The first phase of the descent from the peak can, however, be continued as a straight line, and where it cuts the abscissa gives the duration of the first passage of the dye through the artery. The mean concentration of the dye in the arterial blood during this time can be obtained from the area under the curve.

In the experiment at rest (solid line in Fig. 13.1a) the mean concentration of dye was 1.6 mg/l during the first circulation time of 39 s. The volume containing the 5 mg injected must therefore have been 5/1.6 = 3.1 l. This volume took 39 s to pass the sampling point, so in 1 min the flow (= cardiac output) would have been 3.1 × 60/39 = 4.77 l/min.

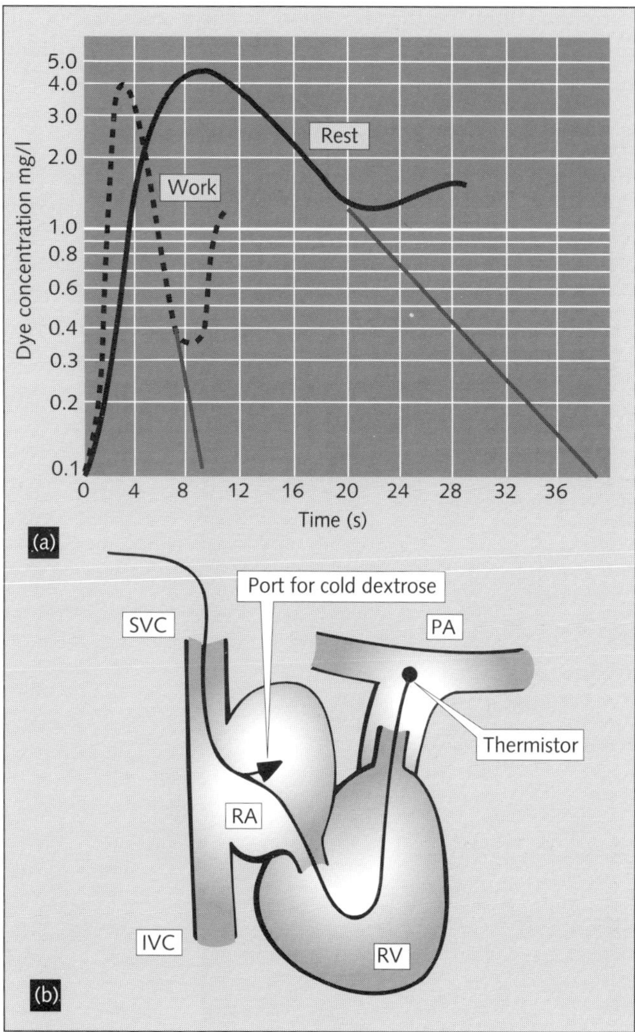

Figure 13.1
(a) Dye dilution experiments to measure cardiac output. Dye concentration curves for the rest experiment (solid line = cardiac output 4.73 l/min) and for the work experiment (dashed line = cardiac output 21.9 l/min). The calculations are described in the text. (b) Sketch of the catheter in position for thermal dilution measurement of heart output. SVC, IVC, superior and inferior venae cavae; RA, RV, right atrium and ventricle; PA, pulmonary artery.

In the experiment in which work was done, the time for the first passage of the substance through the artery where the sampling was taking place was 9 s, the mean concentration of the substance in the blood was 1.5 mg/l and the cardiac output was 21.9 l/min.

Dye dilution methods can also give indications of the nature of congenital cardiac septal defects: for example, a shunt from right to left heart will cause a hump on the ascending limb of the dye dilution curve as some of the labelled blood takes a short cut to the sampling site without going through the pulmonary circuit.

13.1 Thermal dilution method

Instead of using the dilution of a dye, it is safer and more convenient to use the dilution of heat (or more usually negative heat, i.e. cold) to measure cardiac output. The principle is the same as that for the dye dilution method.

A Swan–Ganz catheter is inserted into a vein and advanced so that its injection port is in the right atrium and a recording thermistor at its tip is in the pulmonary artery, as shown in Fig. 13.1b. Ten ml of ice cold dextrose solution is injected into the right atrium as a bolus. This mixes with and cools the blood, causing a drop in temperature at the thermistor in the pulmonary artery. Cardiac output is calculated from the total amount of cold injected divided by the amount of cooling and the time taken for it to pass the thermistor.

This technique has the further advantage that the indicator (cold) dissipates rapidly and so measurements can be repeated in quick succession.

14 The cardiac environment: effects of altered ion concentrations on the heart

14.1 Introduction

Maintenance of the correct ionic environment is essential for the efficient working of cardiac cells. This is emphasized by considering the effects on cardiac muscle of alterations in the external concentrations of individual ions. Correct pH is particularly important for the efficient working of the contractile proteins as well as for numerous other intracellular processes; it is becoming clear that there are several different membrane proteins which transport or exchange H^+ ions to minimize pH alterations. Much effort has been applied in recent years to the development of suitable solutions for the optimal preservation of donor hearts for transplantation.

14.2 Effects of alterations of external Ca^{2+}, K^+ and Na^+ ions on the heart

14.2.1 Calcium ions

The entry of external calcium is, as discussed in Chapter 10, essential for excitation–contraction coupling in cardiac muscle, as can be readily demonstrated by perfusing an isolated frog heart with a solution of salts (Ringer's solution) lacking calcium ions (Fig. 10.1). Clinically, low and high plasma calcium levels will cause weak or excessively strong cardiac contractions, respectively. However, clinical syndromes associated with abnormal calcium levels are dominated by effects outside the heart.

14.2.2 Potassium

Raised external potassium concentration depolarizes all excitable cells according to the Nernst equation (Chapter 4). The depolarization inactivates sodium channels so that at high levels of external potassium the upstroke of the ventricular action potential is largely or wholly carried by inward calcium current ($i_{Ca,L}$). Such action potentials are also much shorter than normal ones, largely because of the properties of the ventricular potassium currents which increase when the resting potential is depolarized and thus repolarize the membrane earlier than normal (Fig. 14.1). Such action potentials propagate more slowly through the myocardium than do normal ones and are also much reduced in duration. Slow propagation and shortened refractory period are both arrhythmogenic factors (see Chapter 7) and the short action potentials give rise to briefer, weaker contractions.

Plasma K^+ concentrations of 8 mmol/l and above can lead to life-threatening arrhythmias in subjects at rest. The high external potassium seen in exercise does not, however, cause arrhythmias in healthy subjects. An important protective factor is the high level of catecholamines in exercise which greatly augments $i_{Ca,L}$ (see Chapter 12). This increases the upstroke and duration of the cardiac action potentials, counteracting the tendency to arrhythmia. This protective effect of adrenaline is shown in Fig. 14.2 where an isolated perfused rabbit heart was subjected to a doubling of external potassium concentration ($[K^+]_o$) (to 8 mmol/l from the normal 4 mmol/l) with consequent loss of output pressure and electrocardiogram (ECG) changes. Further increase in $[K^+]_o$ was accompanied by addition of 80 nmol/l adrenaline, and instead of further decline, the output pressure recovered and the ECG was restored to near normal.

As shown in the records in Fig. 14.2, high external potassium causes characteristic changes in the ECG which can be useful diagnostically. The P waves become difficult to identify, the ST segment is not clearly defined and the T waves are large and peaked.

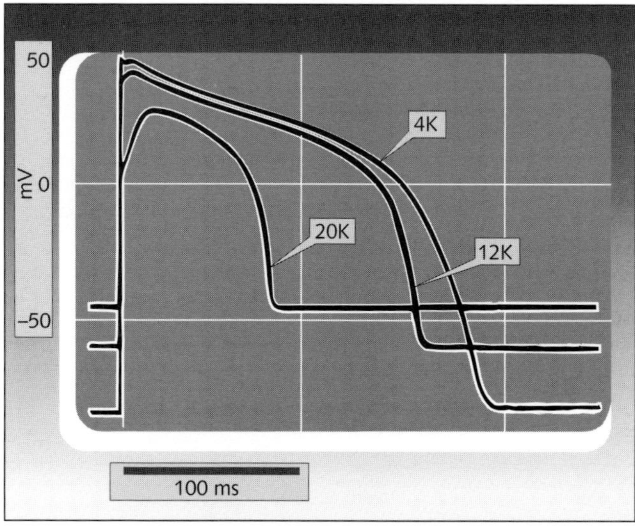

Figure 14.1
Action potentials recorded from a guinea-pig ventricular myocyte in different external concentrations of potassium: 4, 12 and 20 mmol/l.

Low external potassium concentrations can also produce arrhythmic beating. The action potential duration increases greatly giving long QT intervals in the ECG and flattened T waves (Fig. 14.3). Since ventricular action potentials lengthen more than do those of atrial muscle, atrioventricular block can develop. In low potassium, the Na/K pump is depressed, so that sodium ions accumulate within the cells. The sodium gradient across the membrane is thus reduced and this leads to reduced Na/Ca exchange, with a resulting secondary rise of internal calcium concentration. This, together with the lengthened action potentials, accounts for the greatly increased ventricular contractions that are seen. It can also lead to intermittent bursts of Ca^{2+} release from the sarcoplasmic reticulum and consequent transient inward currents (see Chapter 7) which are themselves arrhythmogenic.

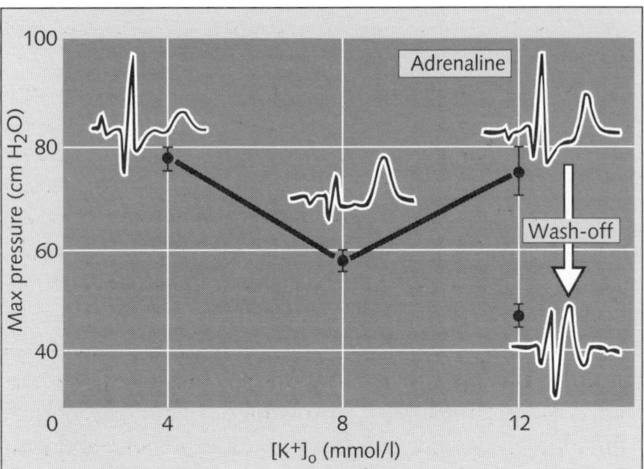

Figure 14.2
The effect of raised $[K^+]_o$ and adrenaline on the maximum output pressure in six isolated, perfused rabbit hearts. Addition of 8 mmol/l K^+ Tyrode caused a fall in output pressure but when 80 nmol/l adrenaline was added together with a further increase in $[K^+]_o$ to 12 mmol/l the output pressure recovered. Washing the adrenaline off (in 12 mmol/l K^+ Tyrode) caused a dramatic fall in output pressure.

14.2.3 Sodium ions

Absence of sodium ions will disrupt cardiac excitation. Lowered sodium concentration leads to a contracture of the muscle as Na/Ca exchange is reduced and Ca^{2+} ions accumulate within the cells. Partial inactivation of sodium channels contributes to the smaller, more slowly conducted action potentials of depolarized cells (see above).

14.3 pH control and acidosis

Optimum pH is important for a wide range of enzyme-controlled cellular processes. A fall in intracellular pH (pH_i) inhibits Ca^{2+} binding to troponin C so that a fall of 0.2 pH units from the normal pH_i value of c. 7.2 can depress contraction strength by 50%. Changes in extracellular pH (pH_o)

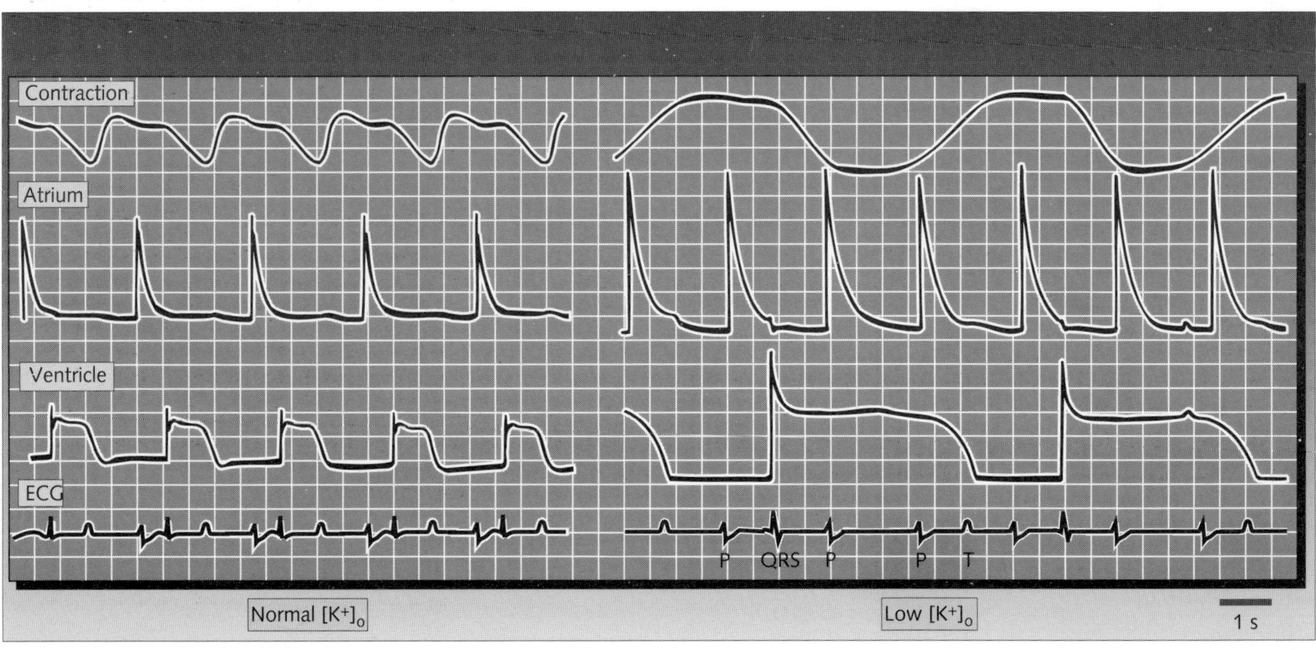

Figure 14.3
Effects of low $[K^+]$ on action potentials (suction electrode recordings of injury potentials) from atrium and ventricle and on contractions of an isolated perfused *Xenopus* (clawed toad) heart.

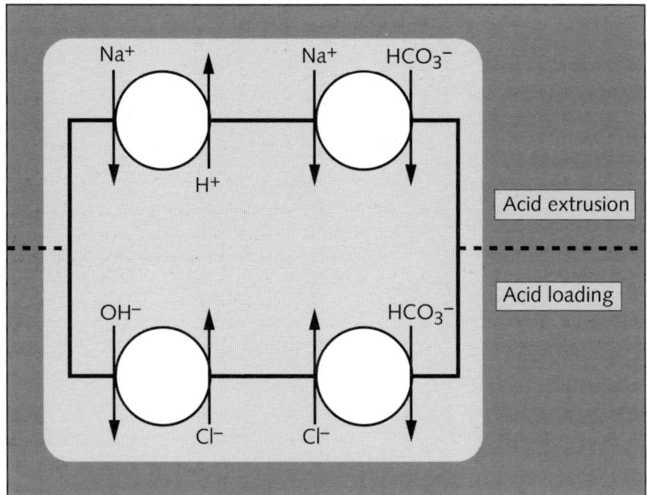

Figure 14.4
pH control in the cardiac cell.

Table 14.1
The composition of the St Thomas' Hospital Cardioplegic Solution.

Component	mmol/l
NaCl	144.0
KCl	20.0
$MgCl_2$	16.0
$CaCl_2$	2.4
Procaine	1.0
pH	5.5–7.5

result from metabolic or respiratory acidosis or alkalosis and will lead to changes in pH_i. Alterations in pH_i can also arise from myocardial ischaemia (see Chapter 15). Such changes are counteracted and minimized by a system of transporter proteins in the myocyte membrane.

The carrier molecules concerned with pH regulation in cardiac cells are first, the acid extruders which are activated when pH_i falls. There is a sodium/proton exchanger which extrudes H^+ ions, each in exchange for an Na^+ ion, and a sodium/bicarbonate symporter which moves Na^+ and HCO_3^- ions into the cell together (Fig. 14.4). The entry of Na^+ ions associated with these two acid-extruding systems raises internal sodium concentration and hence can lead to less extrusion of Ca^{2+} ions by Na^+/Ca^{2+} exchange. This secondary rise in calcium concentration can offset the decrease in contraction seen initially in ischaemia and acidosis (see also Chapter 15).

The second type of membrane transporters concerned with pH regulation are acid loaders which are activated when pH_i rises. A chloride/bicarbonate exchanger removes HCO_3^- from the cell in exchange for Cl^- ions, leaving H^+ ions inside (Fig. 14.4). This is steeply activated in response to alkalosis. There is also thought to be an OH^-/Cl^- exchanger which removes OH^- ions from the cell, again leading to a rise in intracellular H^+ ions.

The activity of these acid extruders and loaders ensures that 0.1 unit of pH change outside the myocyte membrane gives only 0.03–0.04 of a unit of change intracellularly.

It is becoming evident that the autonomic nervous system exerts a detailed but flexible control over pH regulation in cardiac cells by accelerating or inhibiting the acid extrusion processes. β-Agonists stimulate the activity of the Na^+/HCO_3^- symporter while α-agonists reduce it. β-Agonists can also reduce the activity of the Na^+/H^+ exchanger.

14.4 Cardioplegic solutions

Successful heart transplantation depends upon preservation of the donor heart by a cardioplegic solution. This prevents irreversible ischaemic damage (which would otherwise occur within 40 min of cutting off the blood supply to the heart) and facilitates rapid and complete recovery of cardiac structure and function after transplantation.

Extensive research has led to a clinically used method in which the donor heart is first perfused or flushed and then stored in cold (4°C) cardioplegic solution. Cardioplegic solution contains high levels of potassium (20–30 mmol/l) which will depolarize and so arrest the heart, minimizing its oxygen demand. One commonly used is the St Thomas' Hospital Cardioplegic solution; Table 14.1 shows the composition.

Preservation times of up to 4–6 h before successful transplantation have been achieved. Increasing preservation time is important in view of the scarcity of donor hearts and the need for exact tissue typing.

15 | Coronary flow and coronary thrombosis

15.1 Blood flow to heart muscle

15.1.1 How much blood supplies heart muscle?

The blood flow reaching the myocardium through the coronary arteries amounts to 70–80 ml/min per 100 g tissue, rising in exercise to four to five times this amount. Any disruption of the supply is serious and can be fatal. This blood flow to the heart is about 4% of the cardiac output both at rest and in exercise. (In contrast, blood flow to many areas of the body falls during exercise in both absolute and percentage terms to compensate for the great increase in blood flow to exercising skeletal muscle.)

The heart uses approximately 11% of the body's oxygen supply so the arrangements for oxygen extraction within the heart are particularly efficient. Various factors contribute to the approximately 70% extraction of oxygen from coronary blood (which rises to nearly 90% in severe exercise). Thus there is a high density of capillaries within the myocardium, which creates a very large endothelial area for exchange and a short diffusion distance to the myocytes. There are also efficient vasodilator mechanisms in the coronary circulation (see below) and, further, cardiac myocytes contain 3.4 g/l of myoglobin which allows a speeded-up form of diffusion of oxygen (facilitated diffusion) at low partial pressures of oxygen.

15.1.2 Flow through coronary vessels

The right and left coronary vessels arise at the base of the aorta, just beyond the semilunar valves (see Figs 1.2 and 1.3). The driving force for blood flow along them is the difference between the aortic pressure and the ventricular pressure. This is greatest during diastole and, as shown in Fig. 15.1, the bulk of coronary flow occurs during this part of the cardiac cycle. During early systole, when pressure within the ventricular wall is very high, the coronary vessels are constricted and coronary flow remains low throughout the systolic period.

15.2 Control of coronary vessels

15.2.1 Metabolic control

Since oxygen extraction in the heart is already high at rest, most of the increase in oxygen supply during exercise is brought about by increase in blood flow rather than increase in oxygen extraction. Vasodilation of the coronary vessels is caused chiefly by metabolites although their identity is still not certain. Adenosine released by adenosine triphosphate (ATP) breakdown is a contender. It acts on adenosine receptors of coronary arterioles to cause dilatation of these vessels, although there is evidence that it may be most important as a vasodilator when $P\text{O}_2$ is very low, as in ischaemia. Interstitial hypoxia may act directly on the vascular smooth muscle of coronary arterioles to hyperpolarize and thus relax them. Nitric oxide also has a role in coronary vasodilation (Chapter 16).

15.2.2 Nervous control of coronary vessels

Sympathetic nerve fibres innervate the coronary vessels as they do the rest of the heart. Their vasoconstrictor effects (brought about as in other blood vessels, by the action of noradrenaline on α-adrenoreceptors) are overridden in exercise by metabolic vasodilation of coronary vessels. Circulating adrenaline will also counteract vasoconstriction by acting on β_2-receptors which relax vascular smooth muscle. Coronary vasoconstriction can, however, predominate in certain states such as anger.

15.3 Coronary heart disease

15.3.1 Introduction

Coronary heart disease (CHD) probably causes about 1 in 3 deaths in the western world. Inhabitants of Third World countries are certainly not immune, and once the diseases of deprivation are excluded, coronary disease makes a substantial contribution to their death rates also. Such is the prevalence of CHD that its contribution to mortality in the late 20th century has been referred to as the coronary epidemic.

15.3.2 Plaque and thrombus formation

Coronary disease can be defined as atherosclerotic disease of the coronary circulation. It is insidious with a long asymptomatic period before a (shorter) symptomatic period. The hallmark of CHD is the atheromatous plaque. Though uncertainty still exists, it appears that plaques build up when cholesterol in the form of low-density lipoprotein (LDL) passes through the endothelium of the vessel wall and is picked up by macrophages that are unable to metabolize it, possibly because the LDL cholesterol has been altered by oxidation. The macrophages release cytokines that attract other circulating cells into the lesion, some of which lay down extracel-

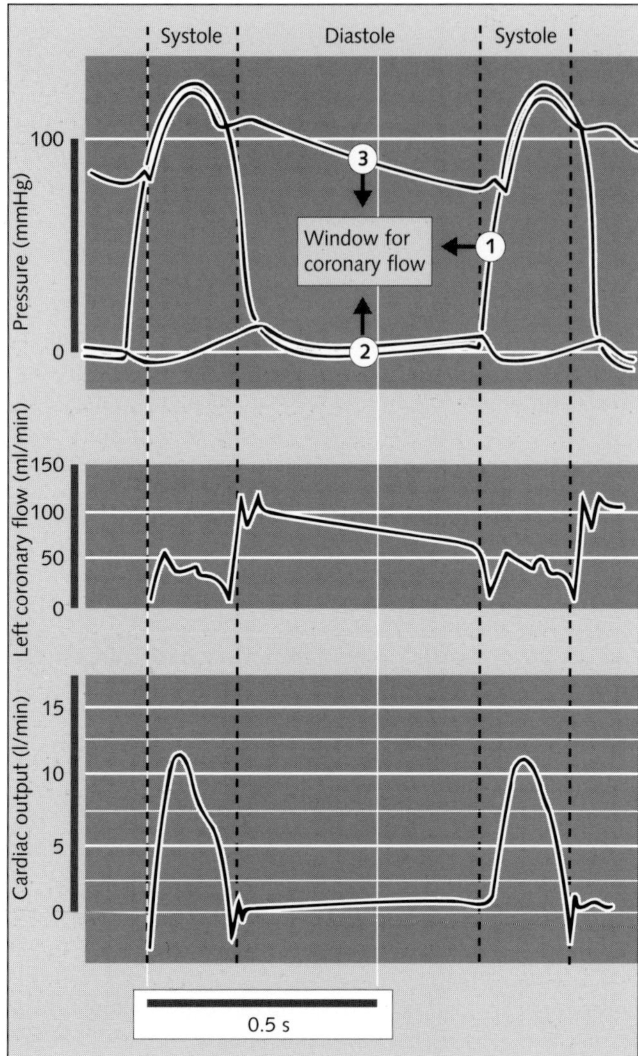

Figure 15.1
Top panel. Aortic, ventricular and atrial pressures showing the window during which most coronary flow (*middle panel*) occurs. This window is reduced if (1) heart rate increases or (2) ventricular end-diastolic pressure rises or (3) diastolic arterial pressure falls. *Bottom panel.* Cardiac output. (Redrawn with permission from Rang, H.P., Dale, M.M. & Ritter, J.M. (1995) *Pharmacology*, 3rd edn. Churchill Livingstone, Edinburgh.)

lular matrix. The plaque may regress at this stage but some plaques do grow, though whether all growth is by cell migration, division and laying down of extracellular matrix, or whether fibrin deposition plays a role as well, is unclear.

Plaques are found in the aortas of individuals as young as teenagers, though in the coronary circulation they start later. In the early years plaques usually grow slowly, and only very gradually encroach on the lumen of the blood vessel, but later on they have an increasing tendency to develop a superadded thrombus which may quickly lead to total occlusion of the vessel and a myocardial infarct. Small plaques can also develop a thrombus on them. In general, small plaques tend to lead to myocardial infarcts, while large plaques lead to angina.

Plaques can narrow coronary vessels to give myocardial ischaemia (see below) and the associated pain of angina. If the occlusion of a major coronary vessel develops gradually, collateral vessels between the main branches of the coronary arteries, which are normally sparse, may widen and proliferate so that they can maintain adequate blood flow even when a major coronary vessel blocks.

15.3.2 Risk factors

Much research has been done to investigate the causes of coronary disease, and over 100 factors have been found to be associated with an increased risk. In practice, however, only a few factors are important.

Age

Risk increases with age.

Sex

Males have a greater risk of coronary disease than women of the same age. Women are protected by the menstrual cycle hormones, and if these are removed by an artificial or natural premature menopause, coronary disease incidence rises rapidly. As women live 5–8 years longer than men, total lifetime risk of coronary disease is the same in men and women.

Smoking

Smoking, particularly of cigarettes, leads to a dramatic increase in risk and this operates synergistically with other risk factors. Cessation of cigarette smoking leads to a rapid reduction in risk such that by 2–5 years after stopping, there is, though measurable, only a small excess risk. There is as yet no convincing explanation for the mechanism by which smoking leads to coronary disease: it may be that smoking generates blood-borne free radicals that damage LDL cholesterol, thus interfering with its metabolism when it enters vessel walls. It may also induce damage through excess levels of blood carbon monoxide. The risk of coronary disease appears to be independent of the tar content of the cigarette.

Hypertension

Hypertension leads to a significant increase in coronary disease. Treating hypertension successfully removes some, but not all, of the excess risk, possibly because many hypotensive drugs have adverse metabolic effects (e.g. increased levels of LDL cholesterol).

Hyperlipidaemia

High cholesterol levels increase risk and total cholesterol levels are correlated with increased risk. Cholesterol is associated with lipoprotein during both its transport round the body and its metabolism. The increased risk of coronary disease is found when concentrations of the LDL form are elevated. The high-density form (density refers to its sedimentation on centrifugation) is protective against CHD. It is the ratio of LDL to HDL which seems to be important.

The rare condition of familial (homozygous) hypercholesterolaemia is a single-gene abnormality in which affected individuals have very high blood cholesterol and a high risk of developing coronary disease in their teens or early 20s. Other polygenic disorders associated with less extreme increased cholesterol levels give an increased risk of coronary disease in middle age.

A genetic link has also been found between increased risk of CHD and abnormally high levels of lipoprotein a, a molecule that has a close structural relationship to fibrinogen.

Diet

Diet, and in particular the differences in national diet, is important. Japanese men have a low incidence of coronary disease in Japan, but once they migrate to the USA, and assume the indigenous diet there, there is a dramatic increase in their rates of coronary disease. The influence of diet is mediated in part through the amount of fat, including the ratio of saturated to unsaturated fat, and ingested cholesterol (see above and Further Reading, p. 121).

Diabetes mellitus

Diabetes, particularly if it is poorly controlled, or in smokers, leads to a dramatic increase in risk. This is partly due to the diabetic condition altering cholesterol metabolism, and partly directly to diabetic tissue damage.

Obesity and inactivity

Obesity operates partly through other risk factors: most obese people have high blood pressure and are relatively inactive and many have impaired glucose tolerance (a mild form of diabetes). As a consequence of such complex metabolic and physiological changes they are more prone to coronary disease and, with any pattern of coronary disease, more severe symptoms.

Other factors

There are many other factors associated with coronary disease, though most are only of academic importance.

Increases in white cell concentration confer increased risk, as do increases in platelets and some of the haemostatic factors.

15.3.3 Prevention

Diet

Much evidence exists to suggest that reducing the amount of fat, and particularly the amount of saturated fat and cholesterol, in the diet can be protective against risk of CHD although it is very difficult to reduce low density lipoprotein in cholesterol by diet alone; drugs have to be used. Certain other dietary factors may also be protective, such as a diet high in vegetable matter. Alcohol in moderate amounts (2–4 units/day) is associated with lower total mortality rates, due to lower rates of coronary disease. Red wine prevents the oxidation of LDL and this may be part of the explanation of its protective action. The amount of solutes in the water (the hardness) has a bearing, with hard-(solute-rich) water areas having lower disease rates than soft-water areas.

Cholesterol-lowering drugs

Cholesterol-lowering drugs have been shown to reduce the risk of CHD. Thus a series of recent large clinical trials of inhibitors of cholesterol synthesis (statins) have not only given a 42% risk reduction in CHD in patients with angina or previous myocardial infarction, but have shown considerable reduction in risk of CHD from reducing raised blood cholesterol in otherwise healthy men of the same age group. Details of the action of these drugs are given in Chapter 16.

Lifestyle

This includes obvious measures to counteract the avoidable risk factors listed above: exercise, which promotes the development of collateral coronary vessels (a minimum of 30 min 2–3 times a week is recommended), avoidance of obesity, no smoking, etc.

Prophylactic aspirin therapy

Aspirin has been shown to reduce substantially the risk of acute myocardial infarction and death in those with established coronary disease. This encouraging result suggests that aspirin may represent a long-term prophylactic approach to the prevention of infarction. Indeed, some clinicians now suggest daily low doses of the drug for middle-aged individuals who may be prone to coronary artery disease. Details of its probable mode of action are given in Chapter 16. Long-term effects of aspirin therapy are being investigated.

15.4 Myocardial ischaemia

CHD leads to myocardial ischaemia or lack of adequate blood flow to heart muscle. This deprives myocytes of substrates and allows metabolites to accumulate, with consequences ranging from transitory localized cell damage to fatal cardiac arrest.

Myocardial ischaemia is characterized by contractile failure though calcium transients can be shown to remain

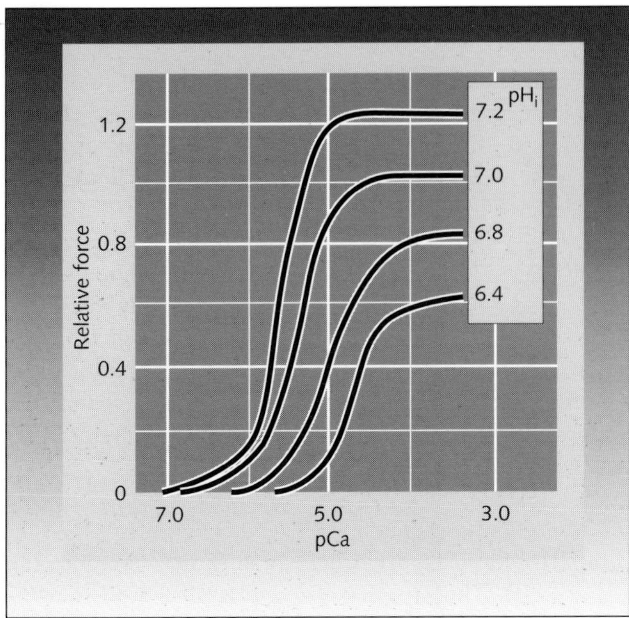

Figure 15.2
Sensitivity of myofilaments to pCa at various pH levels (pCa is Ca^{2+} ion concentration expressed on a negative logarithmic scale).

high in ischaemic cells. There is accumulation of H^+ ions within the cells (amounting to a fall of 0.5 of a pH unit) as lactic acid accumulates when oxygen falls. This acidosis decreases the sensitivity of myofilaments to calcium (Fig. 15.2) so, although calcium levels are high, contractions are reduced. It will also lead to elevated Na^+/H^+ exchange which will raise intracellular Na^+ concentration. This, in turn, will result in lowered Na^+/Ca^{2+} exchange (consequent on the reduced Na^+ gradient across the membrane) contributing to the raised free calcium level in the cells. Details of the cellular mechanisms which control pH are given in Chapter 14.

ATP levels are initially maintained in ischaemia (at the expense of creatine phosphate levels) but then ATP falls. This interferes with many metabolic processes, including the pumping of Ca^{2+} out of the cytosol (into the sarcoplasmic reticulum and across the outer membrane) which contributes to the raised free calcium level. Low ATP levels also lead to the opening of ATP-sensitive potassium channels (Chapter 7) which shortens action potentials, reduces contractions and contributes to the raised extracellular potassium which is a feature of ischaemia. Raised $[K]_o$ will itself lead to depolarization of membranes and shortened, slowly conducted, action potentials (Chapter 14) changes which increase the risk of arrhythmia, as does also the raised concentration of free calcium within the cells (Chapter 7). The period of reperfusion after experimentally induced ischaemia is found to be one in which arrhythmias are particularly likely to occur and, similarly, there is a high risk of arrhythmia in a patient recovering from a myocardial infarction.

Figure 15.3 shows the factors which contribute to myocardial ischaemia.

15.5 Clinical syndromes

There are two main syndromes due to coronary disease: angina pectoris and myocardial infarction.

15.5.1 Angina pectoris

This is due to an atheromatous plaque narrowing the luminal diameter of a coronary artery and decreasing blood flow, causing ischaemia and pain. Often the luminal stenosis is such that blood flow through the coronary artery is only affected on exercise. The hallmark of angina is, therefore, a chest discomfort typically felt as a constriction reliably induced by exercise and rapidly relieved by rest. If symptoms occur only on exercise and have not changed in recent months, the angina is termed stable; if the symptoms occur at rest (when the metabolic needs of the heart are low), the stenosis is likely to be severe, and the angina is termed unstable. In this situation the chances of a myocardial infarct occurring are very much increased.

15.5.2 Myocardial infarction

When a plaque develops a superadded thrombus, the coronary vessel can be totally obstructed. The territory supplied by that vessel, unless collateral blood vessels have developed, will die and the patient will have sustained a myocardial infarction. The patient often experiences excruciating chest pain ('the worst pain ever felt') which may sometimes be felt in the throat and left arm as well. In contrast to simple angina, the pain occurs at rest (or is not relieved by rest) and lasts more than 30 min despite treatment with nitrates. There are often symptoms of intense autonomic activation, with profuse sweating and vomiting. Patients frequently feel they are about to die. Interestingly, the intensity of these symptoms often bears little correlation to the size of the heart attack. Surprisingly, in older patients and diabetics one-third or more of myocardial infarctions are asymptomatic.

15.6 Treatment

15.6.1 Angina

Drug treatment

Vasodilator drugs are used to relieve angina both by dilating coronary vessels themselves to improve blood supply to the myocardium and by dilating other blood vessels and so easing the afterload of the heart and reducing its metabolic needs. Nitrates can be given, some of which give very rapid relief, and also calcium antagonists, potassium channel openers and β-blockers. All of these cause relaxation of vascular smooth muscle and some of them have actions on

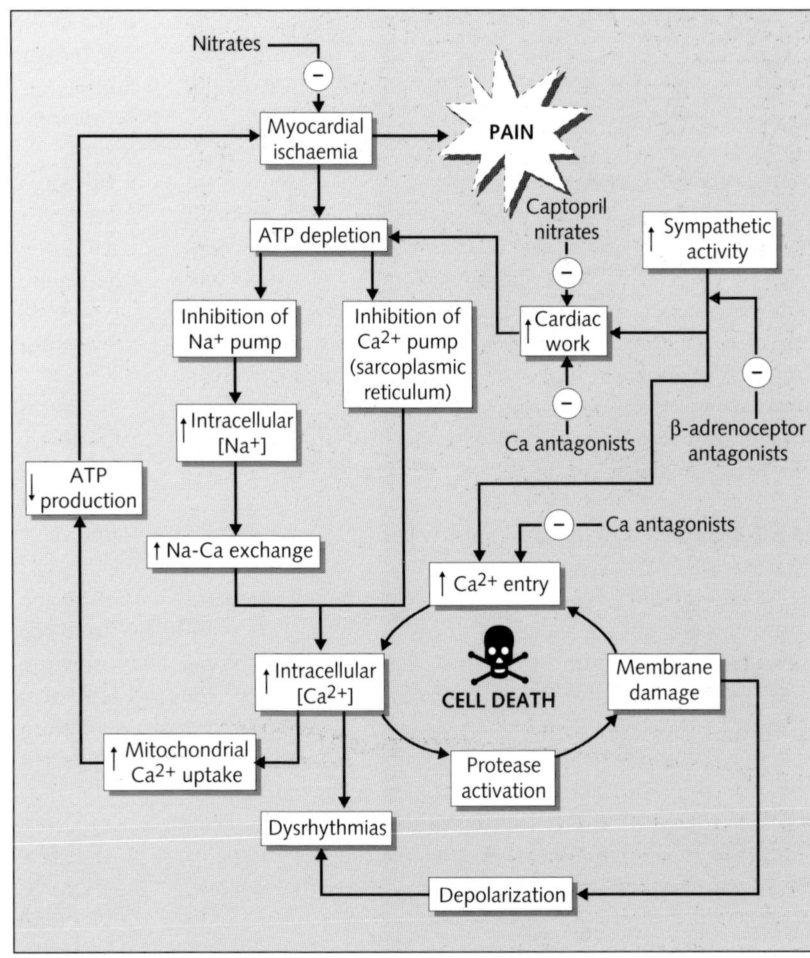

Figure 15.3
Diagram of factors contributing to myocardial ischaemia. (From Rang, H.P., Dale, M.M. & Ritter, J.M. (1995) *Pharmacology*, 3rd edn. Churchill Livingstone, Edinburgh, with permission.)

cardiac muscle as well. Details of their action are given in Chapter 16.

In addition to drug treatment of angina symptoms, it is important to look for and to treat concomitant conditions such as hypertension or hyperlipidaemia.

Other treatment

Non-drug measures can have a major impact in the medium and long term. They include stopping smoking and improving physical fitness and weight loss, which can substantially improve exercise tolerance.

If symptoms prove disabling despite appropriate treatment, patients should be investigated by exercise ECG and/or by coronary arteriography which involves passing a flexible plastic tube, about 2–3 mm in diameter, through a peripheral artery, usually the femoral artery, up the aorta and into the ostium of the left and then the right coronary artery. Radiopaque dye is then injected into the coronary artery; this outlines the atheromatous narrowings when an X-ray is taken. Narrowed coronary vessels can be treated by angioplasty or by bypass surgery.

PERCUTANEOUS TRANSLUMINAL CORONARY ANGIOPLASTY (PTCA)

A small (2–4 mm diameter and 10–30 mm length) balloon is passed into a coronary artery and dilated in the narrowed region to push aside the atheromatous material and widen the lumen. The two major problems with PTCA are first, that in 20–40% the narrowings, after being initially dispersed, return, usually within 6 months and second, that in about 1% of cases the blood vessel blocks off and can require immediate bypass surgery, though the use of stents (wire meshes 3–5 mm in diameter and 8–35 mm in length) implanted during angioplasty into coronary arteries to provide internal scaffolding has made this a less common emergency.

CORONARY ARTERY BYPASS GRAFT SURGERY (CABG)

This process involves connecting a segment of saphenous vein between the aorta and the coronary artery beyond the narrowed, atheroma-containing segment. More recently arteries, such as the left internal mammary artery or radial artery, have been used as conduits. Vein grafts block off at the rate of 8–10% per year. Artery grafts have far lower failure rates. CABG, in selected cases, is very good at relieving symptoms; in some patients with extensive coronary disease and damaged left ventricles, CABG may also prolong life.

Complications of angina

The commonest complication in angina is thrombosis leading to a myocardial infarct. The risk of this happening may be reduced by lowering cholesterol (if elevated) and blood pressure. Aspirin can also be used to lower the thrombosis risk (Chapter 16). The risk is related to the number and site of coronary narrowings which may be estimated from an exercise test. If the risk is judged to be high, angiography should be undertaken to determine if CABG (or PTCA) is likely to be beneficial.

15.6.2 Myocardial infarction

Treatment

Relief of pain and anxiety are crucial first-aid measures, and both can be rapidly achieved with opiate drugs. Drugs are then given with the aim of removing the obstructing blood clot. Large trials have demonstrated that both aspirin (Chapter 16) and thrombolytic drugs (such as streptokinase or tissue plasminogen activator — Chapter 16) improve the outcome if given soon after the onset of symptoms. β-Blockers reduce mortality if given in the acute phase. They reduce the work of the heart and help survival of tissue at the edge of the infarct zone, which has a precarious blood supply.

Complications of myocardial infarction

EARLY COMPLICATIONS

• Ventricular arrhythmias (Chapters 7 and 9) may occur in the first 24 h. These are common and independent of the size of the infarct. Up to a third of those having infarcts die in the first few hours, and most of these deaths are due to ventricular fibrillation (VF). Many of the deaths occur, of course, before hospital is reached. Provided the patient is defibrillated successfully, the occurrence of VF does not have a significant negative effect on long-term outcome.

• Atrial fibrillation (Chapters 7 and 9) is quite common after a myocardial infarction and is associated with more severe underlying coronary disease and thus a worse long-term prognosis. Drugs or cardioversion are the treatments of choice.

• Heart failure is usually due to loss of left ventricular muscle. It is treated with diuretics and vasodilators, particularly those that act by blocking the renin–angiotensin system (the angiotensin-converting enzyme (ACE) inhibitors), which have been shown to improve long-term prognosis. Details of heart failure and its treatment are given in Chapters 17 and 18.

Sometimes heart failure is due to a complication such as rupture of either a papillary muscle or the mitral value, resulting in severe mitral regurgitation, or to a connection occurring between the left and right ventricles (ventricular septal defect) which diverts a significant part of the cardiac output. Both conditions may be correctable by surgery, though the mortality even then is still substantial. The left ventricle can also rupture through to the pericardium, usually causing instantaneous death. Embolic stroke occurs in about 1–2% of myocardial infarctions: a thrombus forms on the endocardium. If the risk is considered high, anticoagulants such as heparin and/or warfarin may reduce it.

LATE COMPLICATIONS

• Ventricular arrhythmias: these can be treated by anti-arrhythmic drugs, or by special pacemakers, including implantable cardioverter-defibrillators (ICDs) (Fig. 5.9).

• Heart failure: the late incidence of heart failure can be reduced by giving those with large heart attacks ACE-inhibitor drugs (Chapter 18).

• Further myocardial infarcts: some estimate of the risk of further infarcts can be made from an exercise test, to determine whether there is early ST segment depression (indicating myocardial ischaemia; Chapter 6) or whether there is angina. If either is present, coronary angiography can determine if there will be benefit from coronary artery bypass surgery. Reducing elevated cholesterol and blood pressure reduces the risk of further infarcts.

16 Drugs used to treat ischaemic heart disease

16.1 Introduction

Drug treatment of ischaemic heart disease aims to increase myocardial oxygen supply while reducing myocardial oxygen demand (Fig. 16.1). Several types of vasodilators are used: nitrates, β-blockers, calcium-antagonists, and potassium channel openers. To prevent or retard atherosclerosis cholesterol-lowering drugs can be given, while anticoagulants help to prevent thrombosis.

16.2 Vasodilators

16.2.1 Nitrates

These are the oldest effective treatment for angina; it has been known for over a century that amyl nitrite and later glyceryl trinitrate (nitroglycerine) could quickly relieve the pain of angina. Nitrates produce nitric oxide which dilates arteries including narrowed coronary arteries, so improving the blood supply to the heart, and having some action on the loading conditions that may lessen cardiac work (see Chapter 18 for more details of their action).

Nitrates fall into two categories: short- and long-acting. Glyceryl trinitrate is short-acting. It is quickly metabolized by the liver into inorganic nitrite which has little dilator activity. It is therefore given sublingually and produces its effect within a few minutes. Long-acting agents include isosorbide dinitrate. Following oral administration this is rapidly metabolized in the liver to the mononitrite which is biologically active with a half-life of about 4 h.

16.2.2 Calcium antagonists

Several types of Ca^{2+} channel have been distinguished on the basis of their electrophysiological properties, molecular biology and pharmacology. The coronary circulation appears rich in L-type Ca^{2+} channels, so called because of their sustained or 'Long-lasting' activation in response to depolarizing voltage steps. Cardiac myocytes possess T-type Ca^{2+} channels, 'Transiently activated', as well as L-type.

A range of chemically diverse Ca^{2+} antagonists has been developed with different pharmacological properties that render them selective for different types of tissue. Clinically, they are divided into two groups:

Type I — Phenylalkylamines, e.g. verapamil, and benzothiazepines, e.g. diltiazem.

Type II — Dihydropyridines, e.g. nicardipine, nifedipine and nimodipine.

The structures of these clinically used examples are given in Table 16.1, where their effects on a variety of cardiac parameters are also summarized. Diltiazem and verapamil are known as type I blockers. They have a pronounced effect on the myocardium and their use as antiarrhythmic agents (class IV) has been covered in Chapter 8. Nicardipine, nifedipine and nimodipine are known as type II drugs. These agents block calcium channels in coronary, central and peripheral blood vessels. Because their actions are mainly peripheral (on the blood vessels) type II drugs are used mainly in hypertension though they are also used to slow conduction through the AV node (see section 16.2.3). Both type I and type II drugs are selective blockers of L-type Ca^{2+} channels with virtually no action on T-type Ca^{2+} channels.

16.2.3 Calcium antagonists

In ischaemic heart disease

Calcium antagonists are useful in the treatment of ischaemic heart disease for several reasons which include effects on the coronary circulation, the ventricular muscle and the conducting tissue. These effects are described below.

Ca^{2+} antagonists and coronary circulation

Vascular tone is dependent upon the intracellular Ca^{2+} concentration. An important factor determining this is entry of Ca^{2+} ions through L-type Ca^{2+} channels. Block of these by Ca^{2+} antagonists will thus reduce intracellular Ca^{2+} concentration which in turn reduces the degree of Ca^{2+}-calmodulin-dependent myosin light-chain kinase activation (an essential step in the activation of contraction in vascular smooth-muscle cells) and causes relaxation. Relaxation of the coronary circulation results in an increased blood perfusion of the myocardium.

Ca^{2+} antagonists and cardiac muscle

L-type Ca^{2+} channel blockade causes a negative inotropic action (i.e. a reduction in force of contraction) and vasodilatation of systemic blood vessels (hence a fall in blood pressure). These effects reduce the oxygen demand of the heart.

Ca^{2+} antagonists and conducting tissue

In the sinoatrial and atrioventricular node conduction is

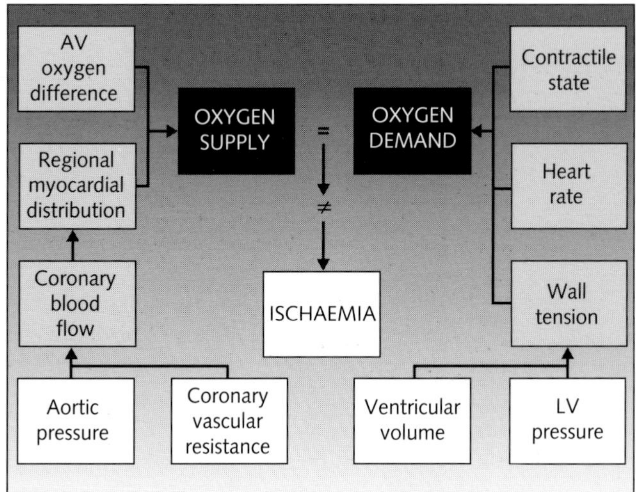

Figure 16.1
The principal factors which determine myocardial oxygen consumption and the mechanism for increasing oxygen delivery. The arterial–venous oxygen difference is always near maximum in the coronary circulation. Widening this difference does not significantly enhance oxygen delivery, but redistribution of regional myocardial flow is of major importance.

largely dependent upon movement of Ca^{2+} through L-type Ca^{2+} channels. The effect of Ca^{2+} antagonists is to slow conduction through nodal tissue. This results in a reduction of the heart rate, thereby reducing the oxygen demand of the heart (see also the discussion of class IV antiarrhythmic drugs in Chapter 8.)

16.2.4 Potassium channel openers

Opening potassium channels hyperpolarizes membranes and this will cause relaxation of vascular smooth muscle. Figure 16.2 summarizes this action. Examples of this class include nicorandil, cromakalim and pinacidil. Of these, nicorandil is proving valuable for the treatment of angina.

The activity of adenosine triphosphate (ATP)-inhibited potassium channels (K_{ATP} channels) contributes to the control of the membrane potential of vascular smooth muscle. K_{ATP} channels are activated by a fall in intracellular ATP and/or by a rise in intracellular adenosine diphosphate and are therefore a link between the energy metabolism and the electrical activity of a cell (see section 7.6.3 and Fig. 7.4). The activity of these channels can be regulated by various endogenous agonists either directly via receptor-coupled G-proteins or indirectly via intracellular second messengers. Their activity can also be enhanced by K^+ channel-opening drugs (Fig. 16.2) and these can therefore be used to bring about coronary vasodilatation.

The membrane potential of vascular smooth-muscle cells *in vivo* is around −40 to −50 mV. Under physiological conditions the activity of K_{ATP} channels is very low. When their activity is increased the membrane potential moves towards the potassium equilibrium potential, E_K, which is approximately −80 mV. (Chapter 4 gives notes on Nernst and Goldman equations which explain this.) L-type Ca^{2+} channels are extremely sensitive to voltage (a hyperpolarization of 2 mV is sufficient to decrease their activity by 25%), so the hyperpolarization brought about when K^+ channels are activated results in a sharp decrease in their activity and hence in the entry of Ca^{2+} ions into the cell. In a vascular smooth-

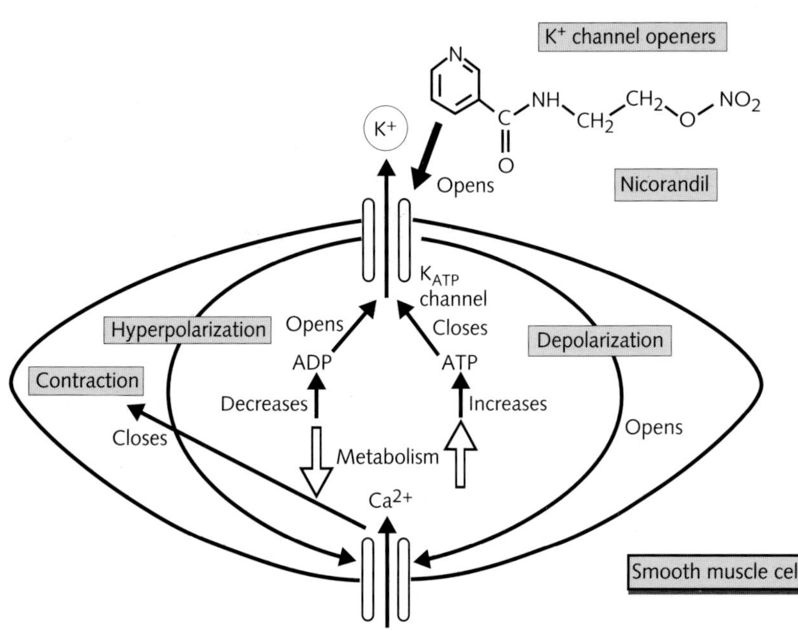

Figure 16.2
Relationship between metabolism, K_{ATP} channel activity, membrane potential and L-type Ca^{2+} channel activity in a coronary arterial smooth-muscle cell with the structure of the K_{ATP} channel opener nicorandil.

Table 16.1
Calcium antagonists used in ischaemic heart disease.

Structure and name	Class	Effects	Usage
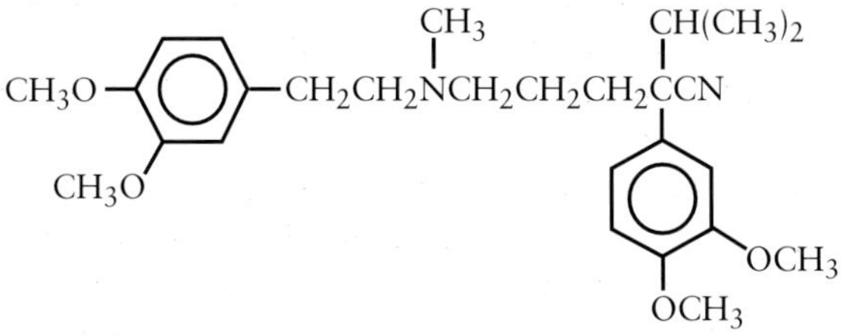 Verapamil	Type I drugs	Marked effects on the coronary circulation causing vasodilation and also depression of cardiac contractility. Profound suppression of automaticity in the SA node and conduction within the AV node	Verapamil used as an antiarrhythmic agent. Diltiazem used as an antianginal
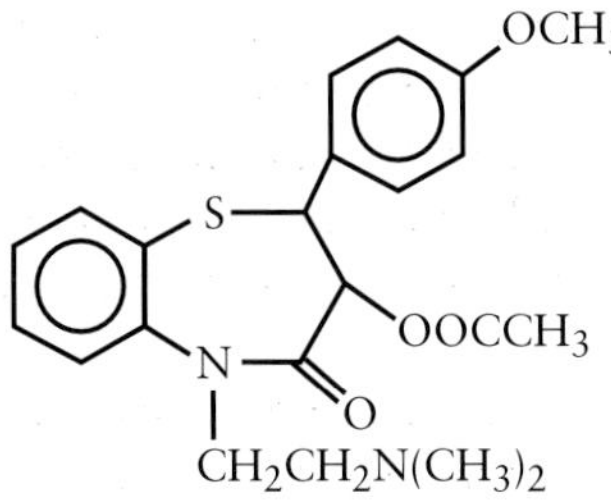 Diltiazem			
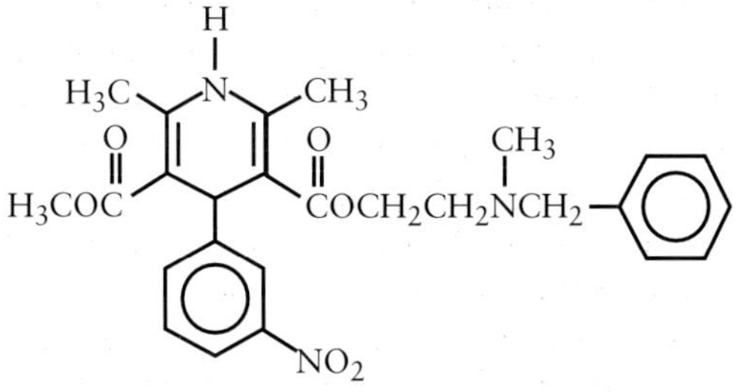 Nicardipine	Type II drugs	Profound dilation of the coronary circulation with depression of cardiac contractility. Slight suppression of automaticity of the SA node with no effect on conduction of the AV node	Used mainly in angina and hypertension
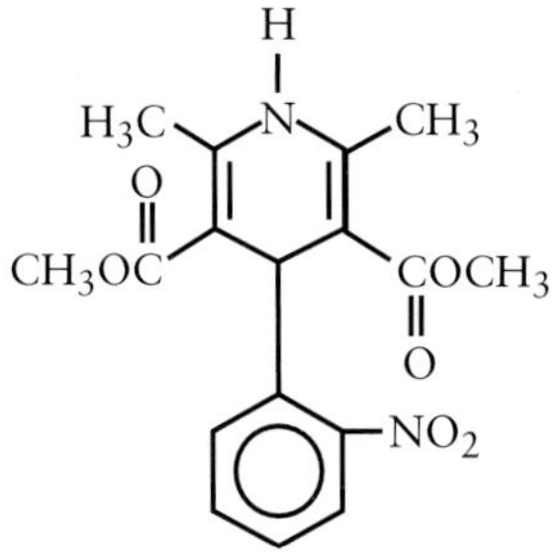 Nifedipine			
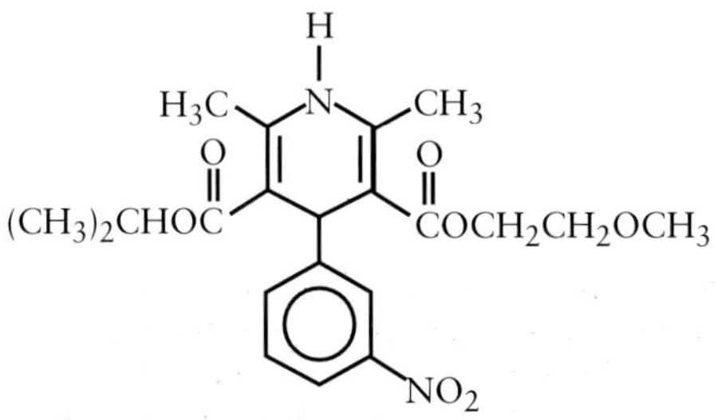 Nimodipine			

muscle cell this will cause a sharp drop in the level of contraction.

Considerable research effort has been expended, therefore, in developing K_{ATP} channel-opening drugs but so far only nicorandil (Fig. 16.2) has proved effective in treating ischaemic heart disease. It causes coronary vasodilation which relieves angina and it improves the balance of myocardial supply and demand by causing a significant decrease in peripheral resistance and reducing both preload and afterload. In addition to opening K_{ATP} channels, nicorandil has a nitrate-like action (see above) which contributes significantly to its vasodilating action. It has also been reported to have a cardioprotective action on the ischaemic myocardium.

16.2.5 β-Blockers (see also Chapter 8 where the use of β-blockers for arrhythmias is described)

Receptors for catecholamines (adrenaline and noradrenaline) are divided into two classes—α and β. These are subdivided into α_1 and α_2 and β_1 and β_2. β-Receptors are predominant in the heart, whereas both α and β receptors are abundant on vascular smooth muscle. β-Blockers serve to antagonize the actions at β-adrenoreceptors of the catecholamines released both from the adrenal medulla and from noradrenergic sympathetic nerve terminals and thus they lessen the heart rate at rest and, especially, in exercise. β-Blockers are thought to have no effect on the coronary heart vessels (indeed, they may cause a slight constriction).

β-Blockers are routinely used in the treatment of hypertension and cardiac arrhythmia (Chapter 8) to antagonize the effects of sympathetic nerve stimulation (Chapter 12). They are also useful in angina as they reduce cardiac work and also myocardial oxygen demand. β-Blockers also decrease the incidence of sudden death and reinfarction following a myocardial infarct.

Many pharmacologically diverse β-blockers have been developed. Atenolol and metoprolol are now the β-blockers commonly used for angina (as well as for arrhythmias, see Chapter 8 and Fig. 8.2). They are both relatively β_1 selective (cardioselective) antagonists and give fewer side effects such as bronchospasm (especially important for asthmatics), vivid dreams, tiredness and fatigue than do other β-blockers, some of which are also shown in Table 16.2.

16.3 Cholesterol-lowering drugs

Among major risk factors in ischaemic heart disease are elevated levels of plasma cholesterol which has been found to be a major lipid component of atherosclerotic plaques (see also section 15.3.2). Cholesterol is derived from both dietary intake and synthesis in the liver; its metabolism is complex. Cholesterol is transported in the blood in association with lipoproteins of different densities which serve to transport water-insoluble lipids in the blood.

Low density lipoprotein (LDL) has been associated with ischaemic heart disease while high density lipoprotein (HDL) appears to have a protective action. There is also a third type, very low density lipoprotein (VLDL).

One line of therapy for ischaemic heart disease is to prevent the development of atherosclerotic plaques in the coronary circulation by reducing the level of lipids (triglycerides produced by enterocytes from absorbed lipids) and lipoproteins in the blood. The types of drugs used for this purpose are described below and summarized in Table 16.3.

16.3.1 Cholestyramine

This group comprises ionic-exchange resins which bind bile salts by exchanging a Cl^- ion for negatively charged bile salts. As the resins are not absorbed, their net effect is to promote bile excretion. This causes a reduction in their reabsorption (into the liver via the hepatic portal circulation) and results in an increased conversion of cholesterol into bile salts.

16.3.2 Clofibrate, gemfibrozil and fenofibrate

These are fibric acid derivatives which lower LDL cholesterol by activation of lipoprotein lipase, which plays an important role in the production of LDL.

16.3.3 Lovastatin and simvastatin

3-Hydroxy-3-methoxyglutaryl coenzyme A (HMGCoA) is a rate-limiting step in the hepatic synthesis of cholesterol. Inhibition of HMGCoA enzyme activity by lovastatin and related agents such as simvastatin and pravastatin, serves to increases LDL cholesterol uptake by the liver. The use of these drugs in clinical practice has increased dramatically since the results of two major multicentre trials (the Scandinavian Simvastatin Survival Study—the 4S study—and the West of Scotland Primary Prevention Study—the WOSCOP study) demonstrated their benefit.

16.3.4 Nicotinic acid

This is a potent inhibitor of LDL and VLDL formation. This is achieved via a diverse range of effects which include an inhibitory effect on lipolysis, a decreased delivery of free fatty acids to the liver, a decrease in triglyceride synthesis and VLDL triglyceride transport.

The encouraging results of trials of lipid-lowering agents in prevention of ischaemic heart disease have been mentioned in Chapter 15.

16.4 Aspirin

The formation of thrombi is often associated with atheromatous plaques. This is largely because atheromas represent a thrombogenic surface which promotes platelet adhesion and further platelet activation and aggregation. Formation of

Table 16.2
Pharmacological profile of the more common β-blockers.

Drug	β-Selectivity	Intrinsic sympatho-mimetic activity	Membrane-stabilizing action	Major route of elimination	Lipid solubility	Oral bioavail-ability (%)
Atenolol* 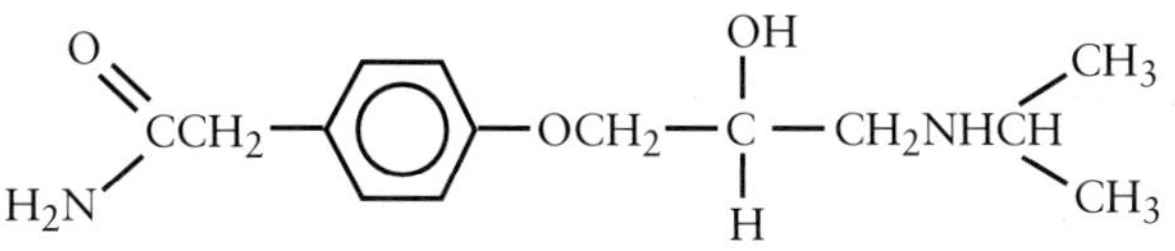	β_1	–	–	Kidney	None	~50
Acebutolol 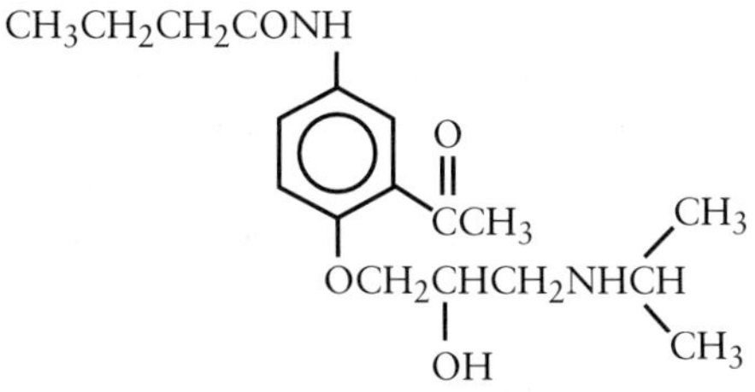	β_1	++	+	Liver	++	~40
Labetalol 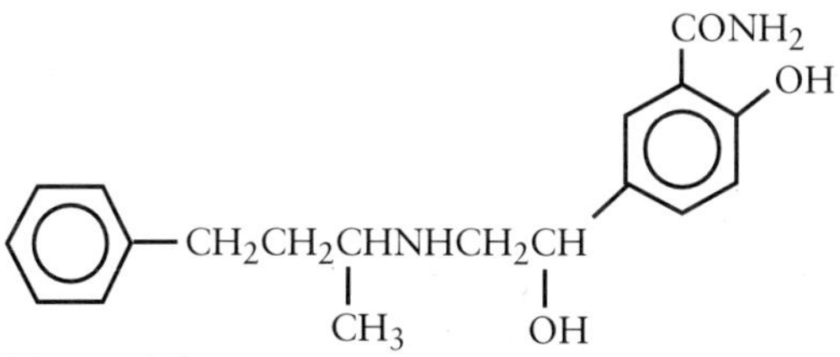	β_1 and β_2	–	+	Liver	–	~20
Metoprolol* 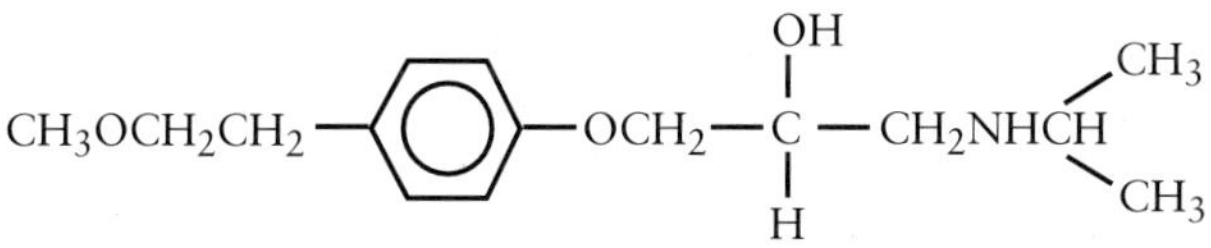	β_1	–	+	Liver	++	~40
Nadolol 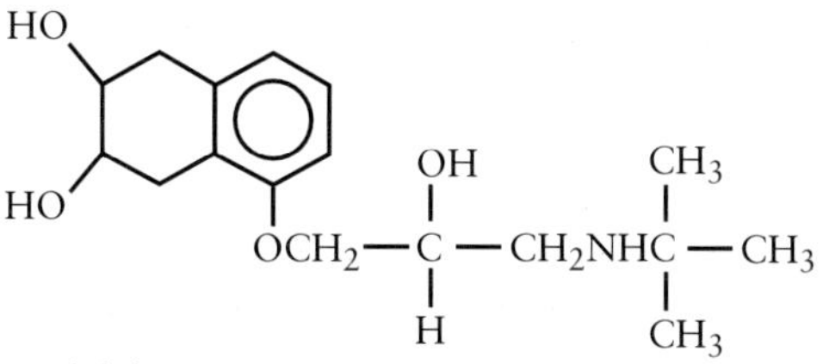	β_1 and β_2	–	–	Kidney	+	~35
Pindolol 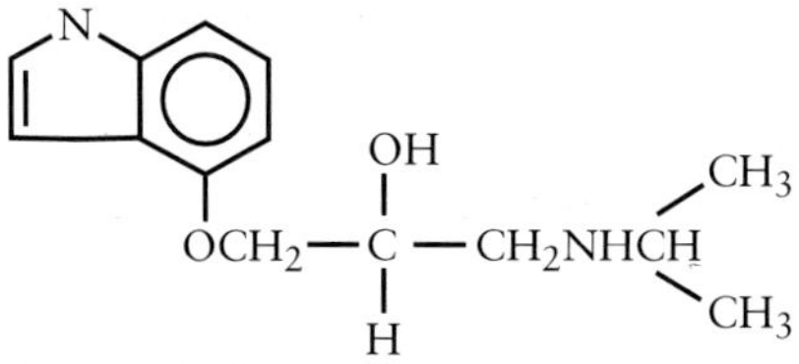	β_1 and β_2	++	+	Liver	++	~75
Propranolol* 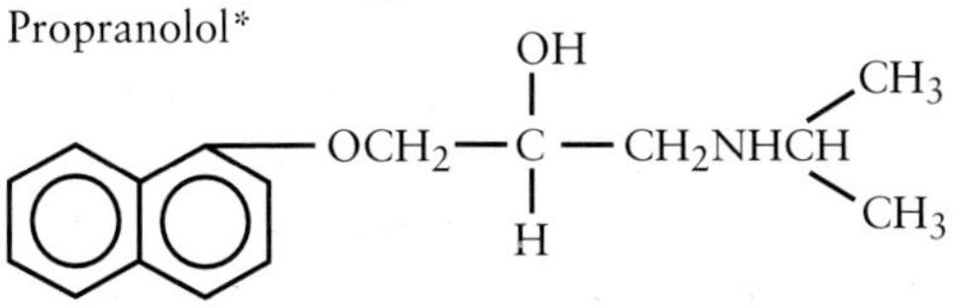	β_1 and β_2	–	+	Liver	+++	~25

* These three are also in common clinical use as antiarrhythmics (see Fig. 8.2).

Table 16.3
Summary of the actions of lipid-lowering drugs.

Drug	Low-density lipoproteins	High-density lipoproteins	Triglycerides	Structure
Cholestyramine	↓	→	→	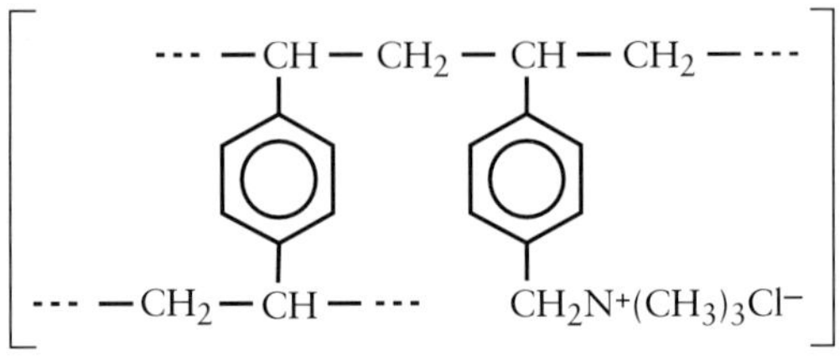
Clofibrate	→	↑	↓	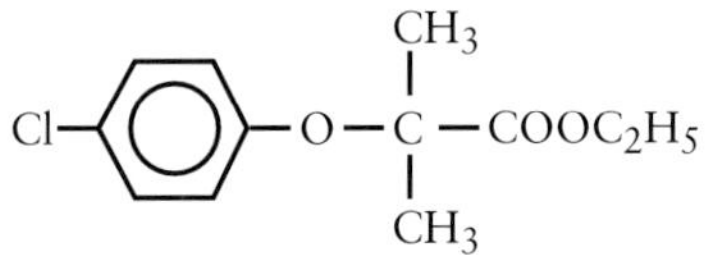
Gemfibrozil	↓	↑	↓	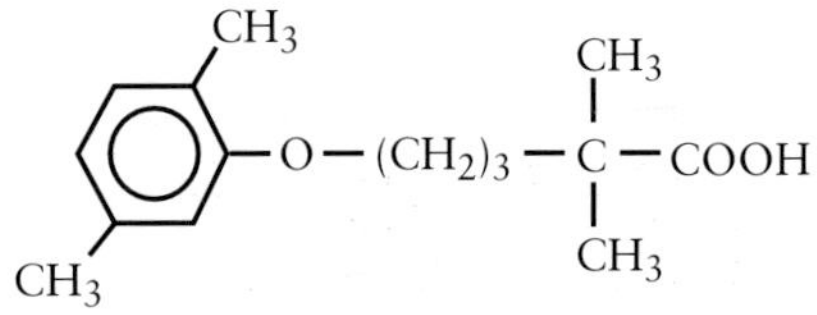
Lovastatin	↓↓	↑	→	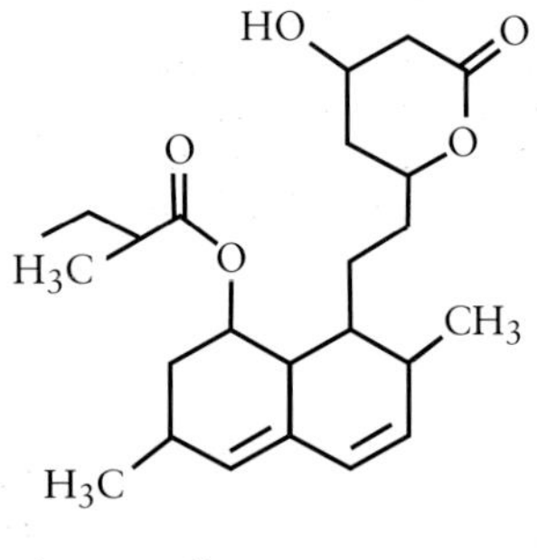
Nicotinic acid	↓	↑	↓	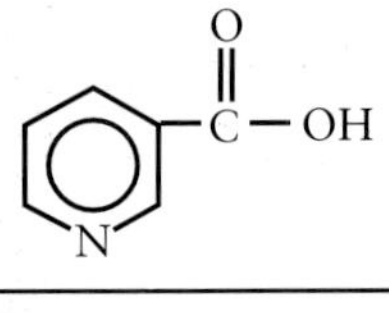

thrombi can lead to either partial or total coronary occlusion and its consequences (Chapter 15).

Aspirin (Fig. 16.3) irreversibly inhibits the enzyme cyclooxygenase which converts arachidonic acid, a membrane fatty acid, to endoperoxides (PGG_2 and PGH_2). These are subsequently converted by prostaglandin isomerase to prostaglandins (e.g. PGE_2 and PGD_2), by thromboxane synthase to thromboxane A_2 (TxA_2) and by prostacyclin synthase to prostacyclin (PGI_2).

TxA_2 is a powerful inducer of platelet aggregation through a mechanism mediated by inositol triphosphate release and elevation of intracellular Ca^{2+}. PGI_2, on the other hand, serves to reduce platelet aggregation through a mechanism involving elevation of intracellular levels of cyclic adenosine monophosphate. Platelets are unable to synthesize new cyclooxygenase while the vascular endothelial cells can. When taken on alternate days, aspirin can produce a selective inhibition of platelet cyclooxygenase. This shifts the balance of the pro- and antiaggregatory effects of TxA_2 and PGI_2, in a beneficial direction, thereby preventing platelet aggregation. This sequence of events is summarized in Fig. 16.3.

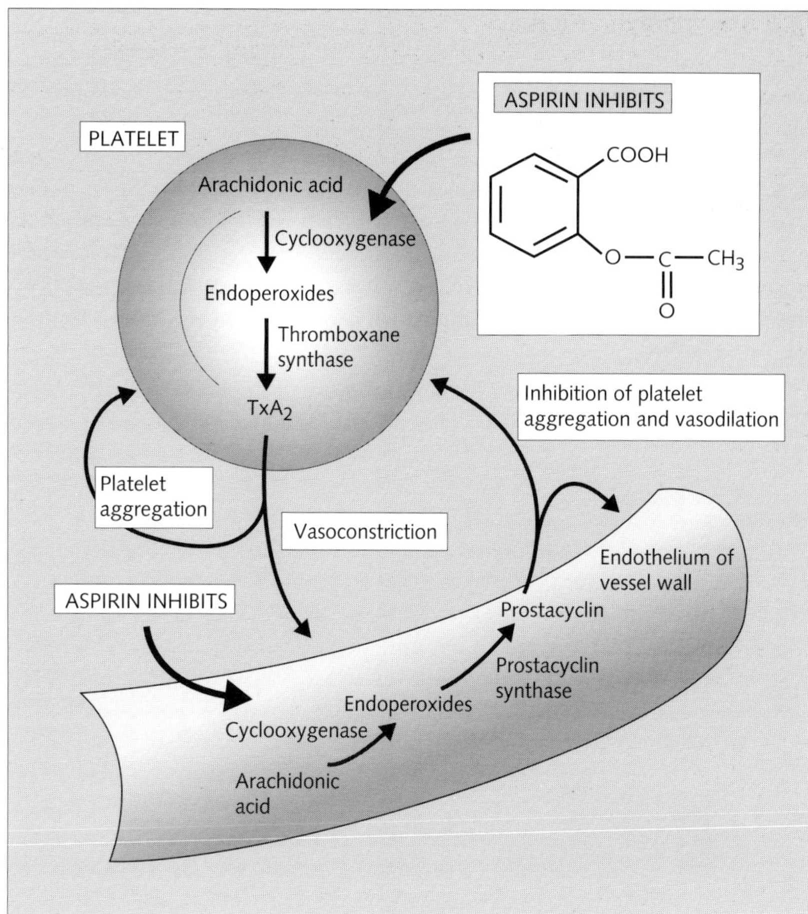

Figure 16.3
The relationship between platelets and the vasculature. Aspirin irreversibly inhibits cyclooxygenase. This results in inhibition of thromboxane A_2 (TxA_2) production in platelets and prostacyclin production in the vascular endothelium since platelets are unable to produce new cyclooxygenase but vascular endothelial cells can. Selective inhibition of platelet TxA_2 can be achieved by careful dose regimens (for details, see text).

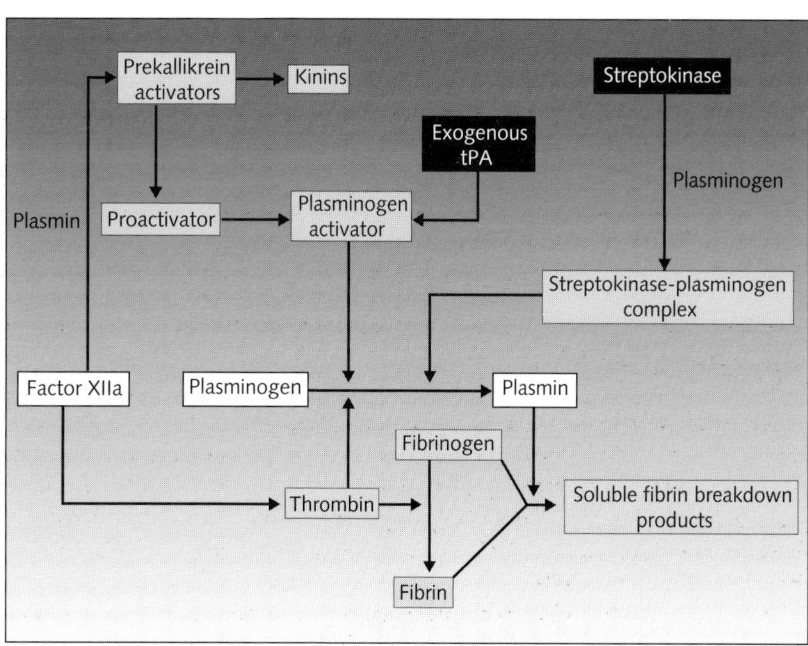

Figure 16.4
Thrombolytic mechanisms and sites of action of tissue plasminogen activator (t-PA) and streptokinase.

16.5 Thrombolytic drugs

The sites of action of the key examples in this class (streptokinase and tissue plasminogen activator, t-PA) are shown in Fig. 16.4.

16.5.1 Tissue plasminogen activator

Tissue plasminogen activator (t-PA) is a naturally occurring plasminogen activator. It is a 527-amino-acid-long serine protease. t-PA binds very effectively to fibrin and activates plasminogen. This produces plasmin which breaks down the fibrin contained within thrombi into soluble degradation products. This agent is given intravenously.

16.5.2 Streptokinase

Streptokinase is a 47 kDa protein produced by β-haemolytic streptococci. It has no intrinsic enzymatic activity but forms a stable one-to-one complex with plasminogen, producing active plasmin which then serves to break down fibrin. Like t-PA, streptokinase is given intravenously.

17 | Cardiac failure

17.1 Introduction

Cardiac failure is defined as an inability of the heart to maintain, at normal filling pressure, a normal cardiac output. The syndrome is common and often carries a poor prognosis. It is often not recognized until cardiac output is considerably depressed and the patient has symptoms.

17.2 Epidemiology

In the western world, cardiac failure is a disease of middle and especially old age, with much the same incidence as that of coronary heart disease (Chapter 15). Women tend to suffer from it at a relatively later age than men. In Third World countries, however, cardiac failure has a different epidemiology. There, many young adults are affected because precipitating diseases are still common (e.g. rheumatic fever), with consequent valve damage and acquired cardiomyopathies, such as those due to trypanosomiasis in Brazil.

Overall, the prevalence (i.e. those affected at any one time) of cardiac failure is about 1% in the UK but this percentage rises dramatically in those aged over 70.

17.3 Causes

There are many diseases which affect the heart and ultimately give rise to cardiac failure. Key examples are given below. Cardiac failure can also be precipitated in those with well-compensated symptomless cardiac disease, by concurrent diseases such as pneumonia, hyperthyroidism or a cardiac arrhythmia.

17.3.1 Hypertension

Hypertension defined as raised systemic blood pressure ($\geq$160 mmHg/systolic, $\geq$100 mmHg diastolic) still remains an important predisposing factor to cardiac failure in spite of antihypertensive medication. The heart responds to chronic hypertension by hypertrophy: there is an increase in size in both the whole heart and in individual cells. Hypertrophied cells, although having an initial mechanical advantage, eventually become poorly contractile. Effective treatment for hypertension (by the use of β-adrenoreceptor antagonists or thiazide diuretics) allows left ventricular hypertrophy to regress and reduces the late incidence of cardiac failure. Hypertension also promotes coronary disease and myocardial infarction.

17.3.2 Coronary artery disease (see Chapter 15)

This often leads to myocardial infarction and hence loss of left ventricular myocardium and cardiac failure. This can occur immediately if there has been a major loss of tissue. After smaller infarcts the heart may dilate gradually over weeks or months and, since according to Laplace's law (Chapter 11) large hearts operate at a mechanical disadvantage, this may produce late cardiac failure.

Coronary artery disease may also cause cardiac failure when, in the initial phase of a myocardial infarct, tissue around the infarct zone becomes 'stunned' (mechanically inactive but still alive), taking a matter of hours or days to return to full activity. Myocytes can also 'hibernate' during prolonged ischaemia (from coronary disease) with no history of myocardial infarction. This results in severe cardiac failure, although restoration of coronary flow as a result of surgery will, over a period of time, restore full mechanical function.

17.3.3 Valvular heart disease

Narrowing or leakage of either the aortic or the mitral valve can lead to cardiac failure. Such damage is commonly the result of rheumatic fever but the aortic valve can also calcify, particularly in the elderly, in those with renal failure, in the hyperlipidaemic patient or if the valve was originally bicuspid. Some people have slightly 'floppy' mitral valves, which leak a little for many years. These valves can progressively leak more, with resultant cardiac failure. Occasionally, usually as a result of infarction, the mitral valve chordae can snap suddenly, rapidly causing cardiac failure in a matter of hours.

17.3.4 Cardiomyopathy (disease of the heart muscle)

Cardiomyopathy is a cause of cardiac failure, of which three main classes exist. Each of these has a characteristic cardiac ultrasound appearance and intracardiac pressure reading.

Dilated cardiomyopathy

Dilated cardiomyopathy is so called from the pronounced dilation of the heart which results in a marked reduction in systolic contractile function. Often the cause is unknown but genetic predisposition is an important contributing factor: up to one-third of affected individuals have affected family members. This form of cardiomyopathy may also result from a previous viral infection, severe and long-standing alcohol abuse or haemochromatosis (where excess amounts of iron are stored in the body).

Hypertrophic cardiomyopathy

About 50% of such cases are familial; there is an inherited abnormality of cardiac myosin. There is tremendous hypertrophy of the heart, often in an asymmetrical fashion, such that there may be disproportionate hypertrophy of the interventricular septum. The myocytes also become irregularly arranged.

Restrictive cardiomyopathy

This is a rare condition in which abnormal elements are deposited in the myocardium. The commonest form is amyloid heart disease in which, as a result of inflammatory disease, protein fragments are deposited in the myocardium (and elsewhere).

17.4 Clinical considerations

17.4.1 Symptoms

The symptoms associated with cardiac failure depend upon its severity and speed of onset. Conditions that arise quickly and cause acute left ventricular failure produce extreme breathlessness (which is much worse when lying flat) and an inability to speak sentences without pausing for breath. Affected individuals are very frightened, feel as though they are going to die and may sweat profusely. If the disease process is more insidious patients may complain of breathlessness on effort. Alternatively they may complain of symptoms due to right cardiac failure, such as swelling of the ankles and legs. In addition, many people with cardiac failure complain of fatigue and lethargy. In advanced cardiac failure muscle wasting and considerable weight loss are not uncommon.

17.4.2 Diagnosis

Diagnosis is established from a combination of characteristic history and physical examination. Those with failing hearts often have signs of fluid in the lungs (pulmonary oedema) or in the peripheries (peripheral oedema). A useful indicator of right cardiac failure is distension of the neck veins indicating raised central venous pressure. Failing hearts have an extra (third) heart sound (Fig. 2.1) heard early in diastole due to an increase in stiffness of the left ventricle. In addition, there may be cardiac murmurs due to valve abnormalities.

The most useful investigation is echocardiography (Chapter 2) that allows accurate visualization of the cardiac anatomy and will not only show how damaged the heart is, which is a useful guide to prognosis, but may also reveal the cause of the damage. Other investigations frequently performed include electrocardiogram, chest X-ray, biopsy for cardiomyopathy and, on selected patients, coronary arteriography (Chapter 15).

17.4.3 Treatment

It is crucial to remember that cardiac failure is often the consequence of another disease process and it is this process which often needs specific treatment. For example, those with aortic stenosis and cardiac failure should be urgently assessed for aortic valve replacement, while those with alcohol-induced cardiac failure should be given vitamins, especially thiamine, and weaned off their habit. The main types of therapy for cardiac failure are described below, while the pharmacology of the drugs used is given in Chapter 18.

Diuretic treatment

The prime symptom-reliever for cardiac failure is diuretic treatment. Diuretics are prescribed in doses customized for a particular patient, and the dose is usually increased until all excess fluid is removed from the lungs or periphery. In acute left ventricular failure it is useful to give supplementary oxygen to improve tissue and myocardial oxygenation, and intravenous opiates to relieve anxiety and thus excess adrenaline levels, so reducing blood pressure and peripheral vascular resistance.

Vasodilator drugs

Vasodilator drugs have been demonstrated to relieve symptoms and to improve prognosis. The angiotensin-converting enzyme (ACE) inhibitors are the most effective vasodilators for improving prognosis, although nitrates (e.g. hydralazine) given with calcium channel blockers (e.g. nifedipine) are also useful. The ACE inhibitors have few side-effects, though occasionally they induce reversible renal failure in those with bilateral renal artery stenosis. A minority of patients notice a troublesome cough.

Inotropic agents

Inotropic agents are useful in cardiac failure. Cardiac glycosides (e.g. digoxin) are used therapeutically. If they are withdrawn, patients often exhibit an increased severity of symptoms but it has been questioned whether glycosides in fact improve prognosis and this is being tested in a number of ongoing clinical trials. Early results suggest that digoxin improves symptoms and lessens hospitalization but does not improve prognosis. β-Agonists, e.g. dobutamine, are also used in acute cardiac failure (see section 18.1.2).

Chapter 18 gives more detail of the drugs used for treatment of cardiac failure.

Treatment of arrhythmias

Cardiac failure results in a predisposition to ventricular

arrhythmia which increases the incidence of sudden death (Chapter 9). Unfortunately, prophylactic drug treatment for arrhythmia induced by cardiac failure has proved unsuccessful. Indeed, it has been found that much such treatment tends to increase mortality (see discussion in Chapter 8). Once patients have developed ventricular arrhythmias, amiodarone treatment is often beneficial. If this is ineffective and ventricular arrhythmia remains severe an implantable cardiac defibrillator may be given (Chapter 9), though this is still an expensive form of treatment.

Heart transplants

If, despite all available drug therapies, the heart failure patient remains severely symptomatic, a heart transplant can be considered. This is only an option for patients less than 60 years old and without other serious disease. Heart transplantation has a beneficial action on symptoms and survival in the short and medium term, although long-term survival is still limited by late rejection, accelerated coronary disease and cancer related to immunosuppression. To overcome these problems, research is being carried out to produce genetically engineered pig hearts which are not recognized as foreign by the body. This would solve the two problems of shortage of donor hearts and immunosuppression (Chapter 20).

17.4.4 Prognosis

Prognosis depends on a number of variables, the most important of which is the degree of left ventricular damage. The prognosis for patients with cardiac failure due to coronary disease is worse than that for patients with a similar degree of cardiac failure caused by dilated cardiomyopathy. The presence of ventricular arrhythmias, even if asymptomatic, worsens prognosis. If symptoms are present at rest, or on minimal effort, the 1-year mortality may be 40–60%, higher than that for many cancers.

18 Drugs used for cardiac failure

Drug therapy to combat cardiac failure is aimed at increasing cardiac output and acts in two main ways:

1 it increases the strength of cardiac contraction;

2 it decreases the work required of the heart by reducing afterload and preload.

The effects of the three categories of drugs (inotropic agents, vasodilators and diuretics) used in the therapy of cardiac failure are illustrated in Fig. 18.1. Their mechanism of action is described in detail below.

18.1 Inotropic drugs

18.1.1 Cardiac glycosides

All cardiac glycosides, of which digoxin (Fig. 18.2) is the most commonly used are potent and highly selective inhibitors of the active transport of Na^+ and K^+ ions across cell membranes. They inhibit Na^+,K^+-ATPase — the Na^+ pump — by binding to a specific site on the non-cytoplasmic side of the α subunit. This results in an increase in intracellular Na^+ concentration and (because the reduced transmembrane Na^+ gradient leads to less Na/Ca exchange) a consequent increase in intracellular Ca^{2+} concentration, which gives increased strength of contraction of the heart muscle. This means there is an increase in stroke work for a given volume or pressure in both normal and failing ventricular muscle.

Excessive increases in intracellular Ca^{2+} may contribute to cardiac glycoside toxicity in which Ca^{2+} overload results in spontaneous cycles of Ca^{2+} release and reuptake. Resulting bursts of inward current associated with Na^+/Ca^{2+} exchange can trigger arrhythmias (Chapter 7).

In addition to having direct effects on cardiac muscle, cardiac glycosides also have a number of other actions on the peripheral circulation beneficial to the treatment of cardiac failure. These are given in Table 18.1.

Cardiac glycoside toxicity

The main cardiac glycosides, although useful therapeutically, have a low therapeutic index (the difference between the therapeutic level and the toxic level). Early indicators of toxicity are nausea and vomiting, often accompanied by dizziness and confusion. These signs often serve as a warning of more serious cardiac side-effects which can be dangerous. Many types of arrhythmia can occur, the commonest being heart block and coupled ventricular extrasystoles. Continued administration of glycosides can lead to ventricular tachycardia and death due to ventricular fibrillation.

18.1.2 β-Sympathomimetic agents

Dopamine and dobutamine (Fig. 18.3) are the positive inotropic agents of choice for the short-term support of the circulation in advanced cardiac failure. Both these agents have inotropic effects on the failing myocardium which are similar to those of β-adrenergic agonists (Chapter 12). There is, however, little evidence that their use improves prognosis. Dopamine is used in low doses to selectively dilate renal arteries to improve renal function in hypotensive patients.

Dobutamine causes less tachycardia and appears to be less arrhythmogenic than the endogenous catecholamines or isoprenaline. Dobutamine also has actions which tend to reduce afterload: it blocks α receptors on blood vessels and so acts as a vasodilator. For most patients with advanced cardiac failure dobutamine is superior to dopamine which lacks this vasodilating action.

18.1.3 Phosphodiesterase (PDE) inhibitors

The intracellular cascade of reactions which link the activation of β-receptors with channel or pump stimulation has been given in Fig. 12.8. Phosphodiesterases break down cyclic adenosine monophosphate (cAMP) intracellularly, thereby limiting the action of β-adrenoreceptor stimulation. Inhibiting phosphodiesterases will increase intracellular cAMP concentration and produce a positive inotropic effect.

Several inhibitors of the type III (heart-specific) PDE family have been used in the treatment of severe heart failure, these include amrinone and milrinone (Fig. 18.4), both of which are bipyridine derivatives. These agents cause vasodilation with a consequent fall in systemic vascular resistance and increase both the force of contraction and velocity of relaxation of cardiac muscle. Unfortunately, trials have shown that the use of amrinone and milrinone in cardiac failure is associated with increased mortality, mainly due to an increase in ventricular arrhythmias. They are currently only used for short periods in very severe heart failure, e.g. in those awaiting heart-transplants.

18.2 Vasodilators

Heart failure is associated with great increases in peripheral

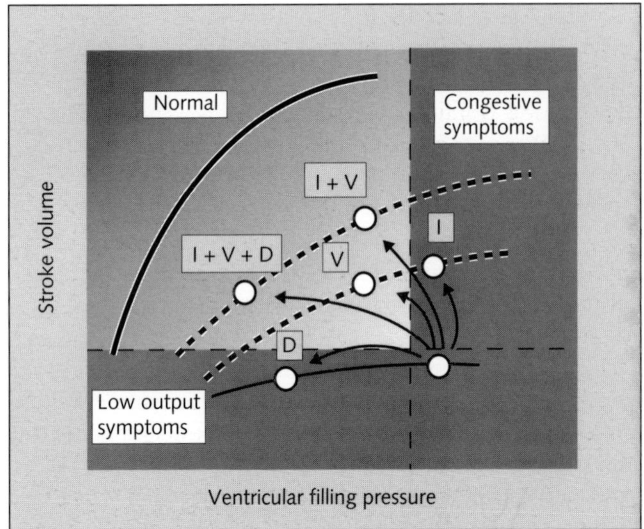

Figure 18.1
The relationship between diastolic filling pressure (preload) and cardiac output for a patient with a normal heart (black line) and a failing heart (hatched lines). Note that positive inotropic agents (I) move patients to a higher ventricular function curve. Vasodilators (V) have a similar effect but also reduce cardiac filling pressure. Diuretics (D) improve symptoms of cardiac failure by moving patients to lower cardiac filling pressures along the same ventricular function curve.

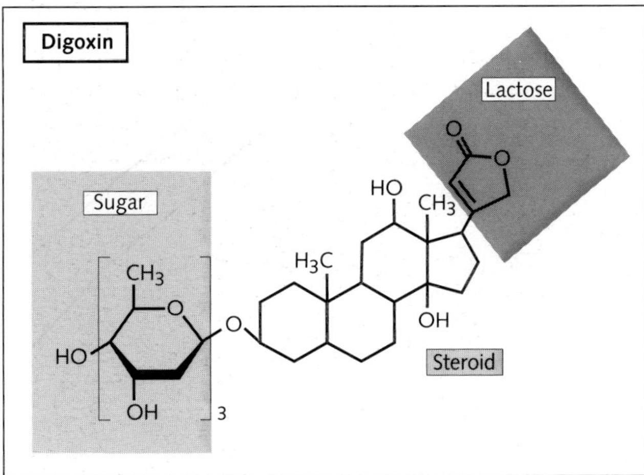

Figure 18.2
Structure of digoxin. All cardiac glycosides possess a lactone ring, a steroid nucleus and sugar residues. These are indicated by the shaded regions.

vascular resistance due to increases in the plasma levels of noradrenaline and antidiuretic hormone and to activation of the renin–angiotensin system.

The angiotensin-converting enzyme (ACE) inhibitors and the nitrates are the most commonly used vasodilators in the therapy of cardiac failure. ACE inhibitors have the additional benefit of increasing salt and water excretion and so reducing blood volume.

18.2.1 Angiotensin-converting enzyme inhibitors

ACE is a component of the renin–angiotensin–aldosterone system, which has powerful effects on the control of blood volume and on blood pressure.

Renin is produced by specialized cells of the juxtaglomerular apparatus in the wall of the afferent arterioles of the renal glomeruli. Renin is released in response to:

- A drop in renal perfusion pressure.

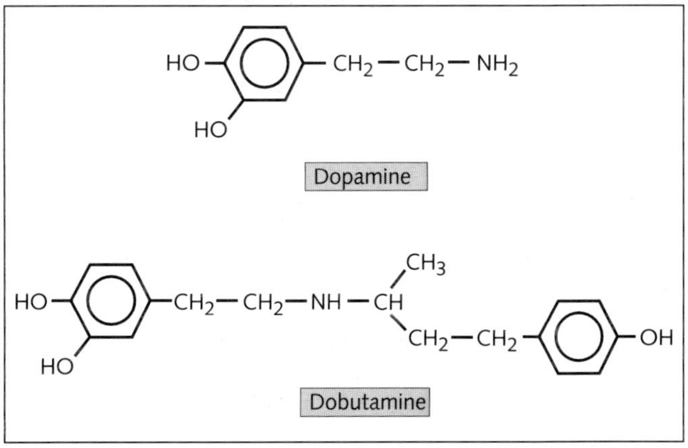

Dopamine

Dobutamine

Figure 18.3
Structures of dobutamine and dopamine. Dobutamine, when administered clinically, is a racemic mixture that stimulates both β_1 and β_2-receptors. The (+) isomer also acts as an antagonist at α receptors, although the (–) acts as an agonist at these receptors. It appears that in human subjects the effects of the (+) isomer predominate, leading to vasodilation.

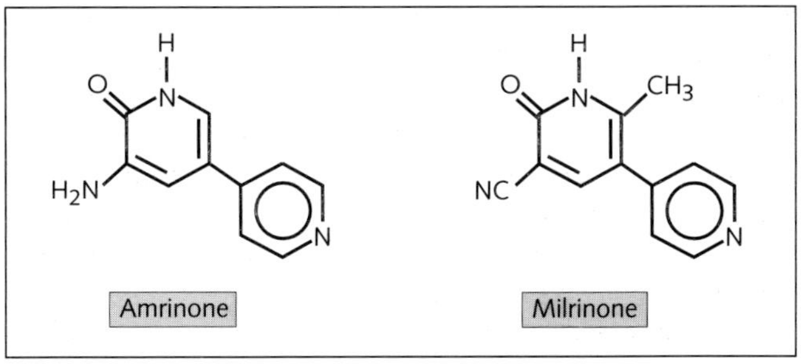

Amrinone

Milrinone

Figure 18.4
Structures of the phosphodiesterase inhibitors amrinone and milrinone. By raising cAMP concentration, these produce a positive effect on cardiac muscle. Clinically, milrinone is approximately 10-fold more potent than amrinone. Side-effects of these agents include hypotension, syncope, arrhythmia and, in the case of amrinone, thrombocytopenia.

Table 18.1
Non-cardiac effects of cardiac glycosides.

Effect	Site and mechanism of action
Vasoconstriction	
Direct	Vascular smooth muscle: inhibition of Na^+, K^+-ATPase and increased Ca^{2+} entry by Na^+-Ca^{2+} exchange (transient effect with rapid administration)
Indirect	
Central nervous system	Area postrema of brainstem: augmented sympathetic discharge, enhanced α-adrenergically mediated vasoconstrictor tone at higher or rapidly administered doses
Efferent neural	Sympathetic adrenergic neuroeffector junction: release and/or reduced reuptake of noradrenaline from nerve terminals
Vasodilation	
Withdrawal of elevated sympathetic vasoconstrictor tone accompanying congestive heart failure	Direct inotropic effect on cardiac muscle Enhanced baroreceptor sensitivity Reflex withdrawal of elevated sympathetic tone
Cholinergic modulation	Prejunctional adrenergic nerve terminal in vascular smooth muscle: inhibition by acetylcholine of noradrenaline release

• A reduced rate of Na^+ delivery to the distal tubules.
• β-Adrenoceptor stimulation.

Renin splits angiotensinogen (a peptide circulating in the blood) to give the decapeptide angiotensin I and in turn this is converted to an octapeptide, angiotensin II, by ACE. ACE is found in high concentrations in the lung so that virtually all angiotensin I is converted to angiotensin II in a single passage through the pulmonary circulation. Figure 18.5 shows diagrammatically the steps in the formation of angiotensin II.

Angiotensin II has powerful effects within the body: it causes vasoconstriction of systemic and of renal arterioles. Figure 18.6 illustrates the outcome of the constriction of the efferent glomerular arterioles brought about by angiotensin II. The constriction of renal blood flow leads directly to sodium and water retention and this is augmented by the stimulation of aldosterone and antidiuretic hormone (ADH) output which angiotensin II also brings about. This increases blood volume, leading to raised blood pressure and increased afterload and preload of the heart.

ACE inhibitors, of which the two commonest are captopril and enalapril (Fig. 18.7), reduce the production of angiotensin II and therefore counteract all these effects.

• They increase vasodilatation, which reduces afterload.
• They can lead to increase in Na^+ and water excretion both directly (by increasing renal blood flow) and through a decrease in aldosterone and ADH secretion.
• Hence blood volume is reduced, reducing venous return which, together with venodilatation, leads to a further reduction in preload.

Cardiac failure produces conditions (poor perfusion of the kidney) under which renin will tend to be produced. This creates a vicious circle which is cut by ACE inhibitors, so that the failing heart can operate under more favourable conditions for maintaining the circulation. ACE inhibitors are also thought to have direct effects on myocardial remodelling, especially after myocardial infarction, though the mechanisms are not fully known.

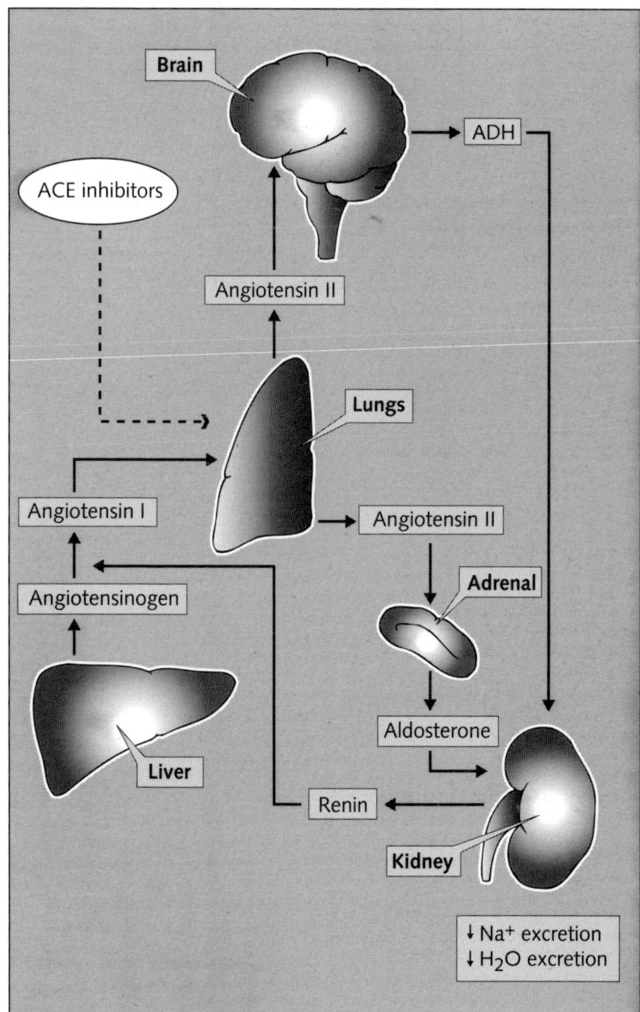

Figure 18.5
The renin–angiotensin–aldosterone system, showing the point of action of angiotensin-converting enzyme (ACE) inhibitors.
Note. There is also renin and angiotensin II production at local sites in blood vessels.

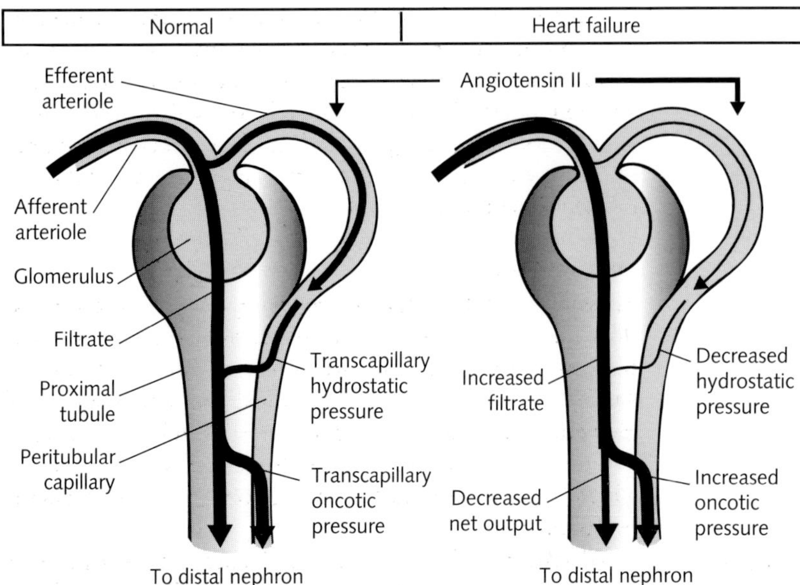

Figure 18.6
In the kidney, angiotensin II regulates the tone of the glomerular efferent arterioles, thereby determining in part the fraction of glomerular plasma that will be filtered at the glomerulus (the filtration fraction). In heart failure increased efferent arterial tone mediated by angiotensin II results in an increase in filtration fraction, increasing Na^+ reabsorption in the proximal tubule. Angiotensin-converting enzyme (ACE) inhibitors decrease the filtration fraction and thereby increase the delivery of Na^+ and water to subsequent parts of the nephron which are responsive to loop and thiazide diuretics.

Figure 18.7
Structures of the angiotensin-converting enzyme (ACE) inhibitors enalapril and captopril. Enalaprilat is the active metabolite of enalapril and is differentiated from its parent molecule by the shaded area. Enalaprilat is more potent and has a longer-lasting effect than captopril.

18.2.2 Nitrate vasodilators

These drugs exert a vasodilating action by mimicking the action of nitric oxide (NO) which causes relaxation of vascular smooth muscle. NO is produced by the vascular endothelium (it was first known in this context as endothelial-derived relaxing factor). It causes the activation of the enzyme guanylate cyclase which converts guanosine triphosphate to cyclic guanosine monophosphate (cGMP) within vascular smooth-muscle cells and cGMP induces relaxation of vascular smooth muscle, although it is not yet known exactly how it does so.

Nitrate vasodilators increase peripheral vasodilatation and thus relieve congestive heart failure. The two most commonly used nitrate vasodilators are sodium nitroprusside and isosorbide dinitrate (Fig. 18.8).

Sodium nitroprusside is effective in reducing both ventricular preload and afterload. It has a rapid onset of action and is quickly metabolized to thiocyanate, which is eliminated in the urine and to nitric oxide.

The predominant effect of organic nitrates such as isosorbide dinitrate is reduction in preload. They are relatively safe and effective agents in reducing ventricular filling pressures in acute as well as chronic congestive heart failure.

18.2.3 Hydralazine

The mechanism underlying the action of hydralazine (Fig. 18.9) at a cellular level is poorly understood. It is, however, effective in dilating both arteries and veins. Hydralazine reduces both left and right ventricular load by reducing systemic and pulmonary arterial resistance. Hydralazine also appears to have a direct positive intropic effect on cardiac muscle. The systemic effects of hydralazine can be so profound that a hypotension coupled to unwanted reflex tachycardia can occur.

18.2.4 Calcium antagonists (Ca^{2+} channel blockers)

These have been detailed in relation to the treatment of arrhythmia (Chapter 8) and coronary artery disease and

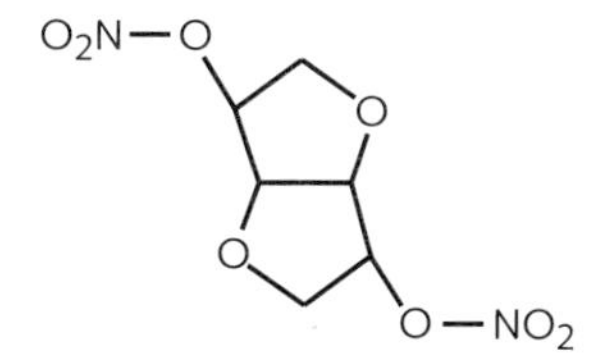

O₂N—O ... O—NO₂

Isosorbide dinitrate

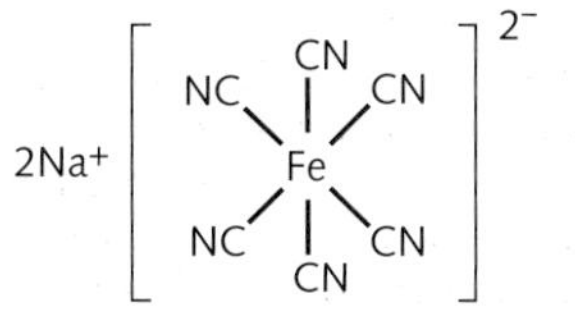

2Na+ [Fe(CN)6] 2−

Sodium nitroprusside

Figure 18.8
Structures of sodium nitroprusside and isosorbide dinitrate. Sodium nitroprusside is administered by infusion to achieve controlled hypotension. Isosorbide dinitrate, which is lipid-soluble, can be applied sublingually, although it is generally administered orally.

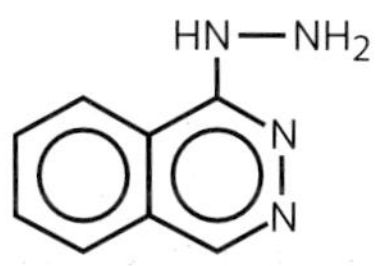

HN—NH2

Hydralazine

Figure 18.9
Structure of hydralazine. This agent is effective in reducing renal blood flow to a greater degree than most other vasodilators and so is often used in cardiac failure in patients with renal dysfunction who cannot tolerate ACE inhibitors.

angina (Chapter 16). Although they are effective vasodilators, calcium antagonists also have negative inotropic effects on the heart and so do not help in heart failure, except where this is due to supraventricular tachycardia or to hypertension-induced cardiomyopathy.

18.3 Diuretics

Diuretics have a central role in the management of cardiac failure. This is because the kidney is the target organ for many of the haemodynamic, hormonal and autonomic nerve changes which occur in response to a failing myocardium. The net effect of such changes is retention of water and expansion of the extracellular fluid volume which serves in the short run to sustain cardiac output but in the longer term exacerbates the heart's problems.

Diuretics act on the kidney to increase electrolyte excretion and hence water output. This reduces plasma volume and oedema and so will increase the efficiency of the failing myocardium.

A detailed account of the action of these drugs is beyond the scope of this text but the actions and structures of the main classes of diuretics used in the therapy of cardiac failure are summarized in Fig. 18.10 and briefly described below. (Classes of diuretic agent not described include osmotic diuretics, e.g. mannitol, and carbonic anhydrase inhibitors, e.g. acetazolamide.)

18.3.1 Loop diuretics

Frusemide and bumetanide are examples of loop diuretics. This type of diuretic is indicated in the treatment of most patients with cardiac failure. Loop diuretics act on the luminal membrane of the cells of the thick ascending loop of Henle to inhibit the cotransporter responsible for the reabsorption of Na^+, K^+ and Cl^- ions. Since the loop of Henle has a high capacity for absorbing NaCl, loop diuretics produce a profound diuresis.

Side-effects of these agents include hyperglycaemia (though this is rare), hyperuricaemia and, if plasma volume falls too far, hypotension. K^+ loss can be considerable and, if loop diuretics are used regularly, they should be given together with K^+ supplements. There can also be loss of Na^+, Mg^{2+}, Cl^- and Ca^{2+}.

18.3.2 Thiazide diuretics

Examples of this class include chlorothiazide and bendrofluazide. These agents act mainly on the early part of the distal convoluted tubule where they inhibit the reabsorption of NaCl by blocking the cotransport of Na^+ and Cl^- ions from the lumen of the nephron into the tubular cells. The major side-effect of these drugs is hypokalaemia since in the later part of the distal tubule the Na^+ is exchanged for K^+. This hypokalaemia may precipitate cardiac arrhythmias in patients also on cardiac glycoside therapy. Thiazide diuretics are used more commonly for hypertension than for heart-failure.

18.3.3 Potassium-sparing diuretics

Examples of this class include amiloride and spironolactone. Both these agents act on the aldosterone-responsive regions of the distal nephron which is involved in regulating K^+ homeostasis. Aldosterone, like other steroids, binds to specific intracellular receptors. The interaction of aldosterone with its receptor initiates DNA transcription resulting in an increased production of Na^+,K^+-ATPase (the sodium pump) which serves to pump out Na^+ from the cells of the distal convoluted tubule into the blood.

Spironolactone is a competitive antagonist at cytoplasmic aldosterone receptors. The spironolactone–receptor complex is thought not to bind to DNA and is therefore unable to initiate transcription, thus preventing production of the Na^+ pump protein. This reduces the sodium-retaining action of

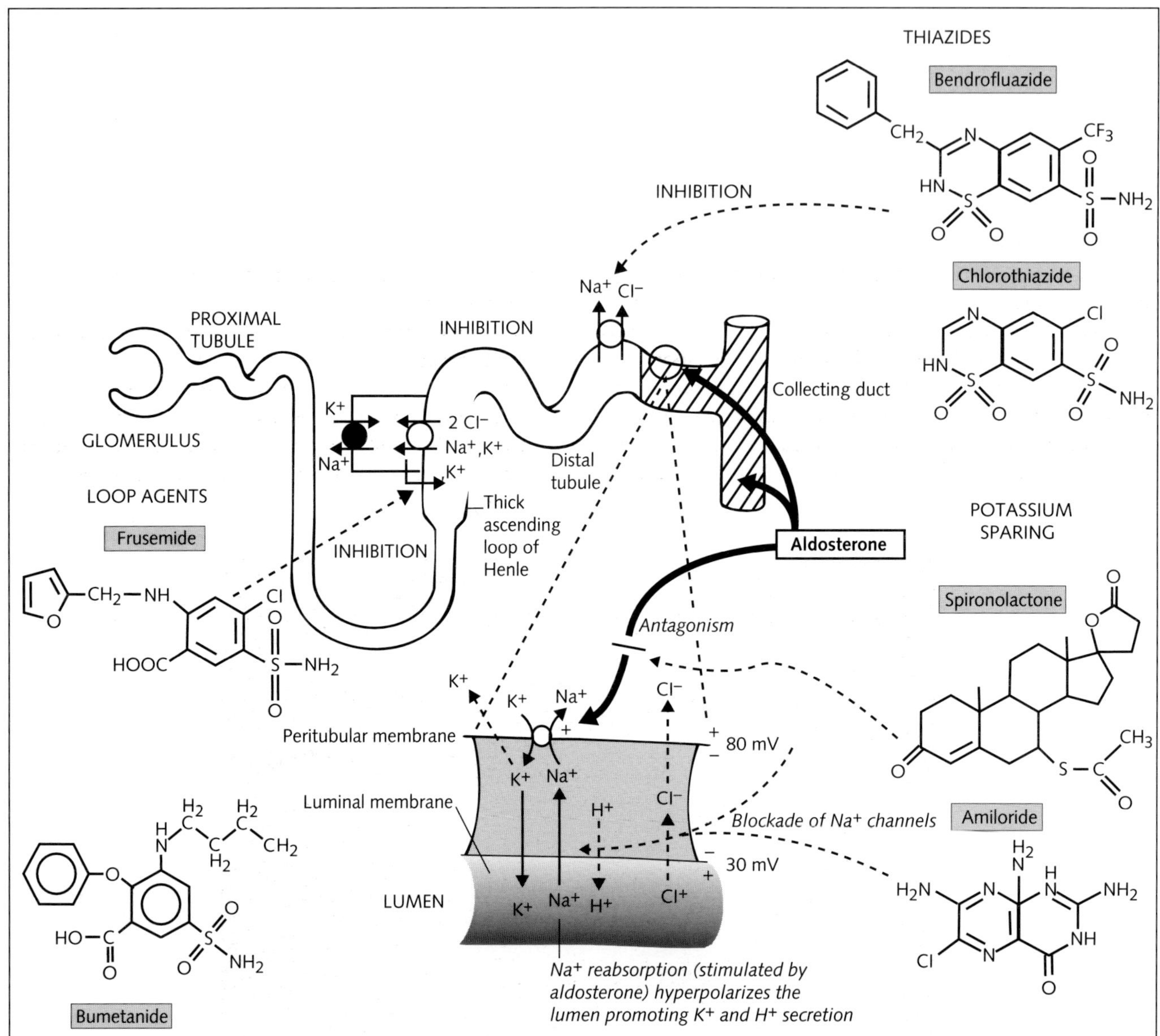

Figure 18.10
Site and mechanism of action for the three classes of diuretic agent (loop, thiazide and potassium-sparing) used in the therapy of cardiac failure. Also shown are key examples of each class.

aldosterone which simultaneously decreases potassium output (Fig. 18.10).

The diuretic action of spironolactone is limited but it is commonly given with potassium-losing diuretics such as the thiazides.

Amiloride, also a weak diuretic, serves to reduce the Na^+ permeability of the luminal membrane in the distal nephron by blocking Na^+ channels. By preventing Na^+ entry amiloride reduces its exchange for K^+ and H^+, thereby conserving K^+ while inducing a net increase in Na^+ excretion (in addition to Cl^- and water).

19 Molecular biology of cardiac ion channels

19.1 Introduction

In recent years there has been an explosion in the use of techniques associated with molecular biology. The discovery of the structure of DNA by Watson and Crick in 1953 heralded this era of modern molecular biology and we may soon be in a position to read a map of the entire human genome. The techniques available for studying and manipulating DNA now pervade all the natural sciences and have major implications for medicine and in our day-to-day lives from, for example, DNA fingerprinting to the start of gene therapy for diseases such as cystic fibrosis.

The cardiac action potential and the normal functioning of the heart depend on the activity of membrane ion channels (Chapters 4 and 5), proteins which also represent targets for a variety of therapeutic agents used in the treatment of arrhythmia (Chapters 8 and 9), ischaemic heart disease (Chapters 15 and 16) and cardiac failure (Chapters 17 and

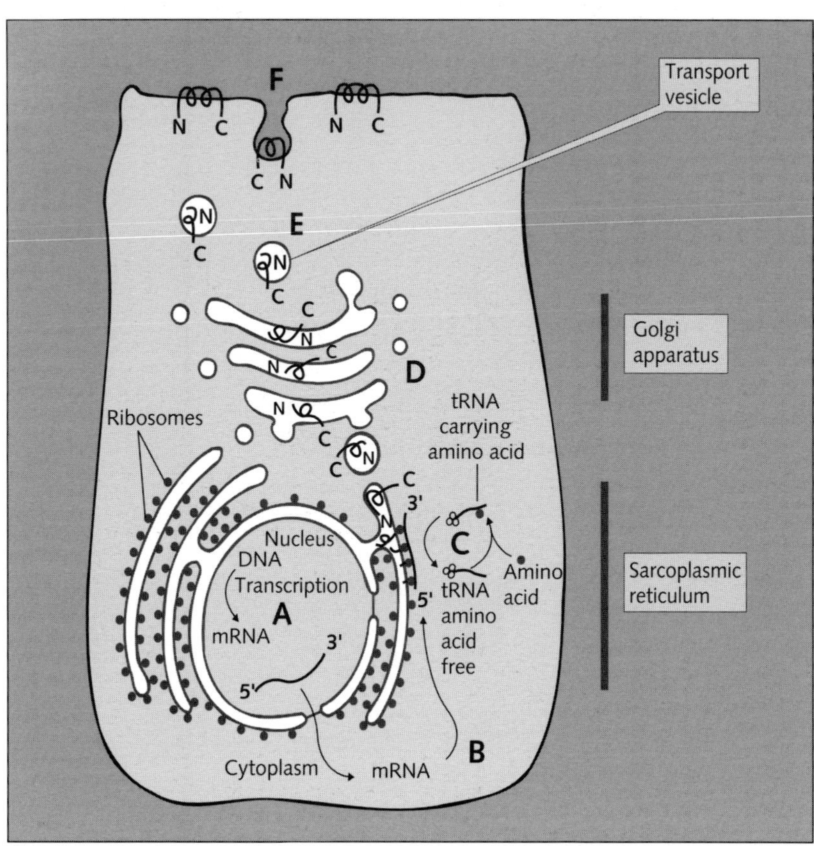

Figure 19.1
Schematic diagram illustrating the synthesis of an ion-channel protein (with C and N termini indicated) and its insertion into the cell membrane. The various stages are annotated on the diagram. A, transcription; B, movement of mRNA into the cytoplasm; C, protein synthesis and interaction of amino acid carrying transfer RNA (tRNA) with ribosomes to form the ion-channel protein itself; D, transfer of ion-channel protein to Golgi apparatus for glycosylation and packaging into vesicles; E, movement of vesicles to the cell membrane; F, fusion of vesicle with the cell membrane and insertion of ion-channel protein into the membrane. It is important to note that stages D–F, although representative of many proteins, have yet to be verified for ion channels.

18). The present chapter focuses on some of the more important molecular aspects of these channels.

19.2 Essential features of ion channels

19.2.1 Formation

Like those of all proteins, the amino acid sequences of ion channels are dictated by the sequence of bases in the DNA of chromosomes contained within the nucleus. The genetic code represents each amino acid by triplets of bases known as codons. These are transcribed by RNA polymerase to make messenger RNA (mRNA) transcripts. The mRNA is then shipped via nuclear pores into the cytoplasm where each codon is read and the mRNA sequence translated into peptides by the ribosomes and their associated machinery for protein synthesis. The resulting channel structures are then fed across the rough endoplasmic reticular membrane into its lumen. They then pass on to the Golgi apparatus for glycosylation and packaging into secretory vesicles which, after their release, fuse with the cell membrane. The process of fusion is thought to result in insertion of the ion channel into the membrane and in this way differs from that of proteins which are actually released from cells. This process is summarized in Fig. 19.1.

19.2.2 Structure

All the different types of ion channel found in the heart are glycoproteins which contain several α-helical membrane-spanning domains flanked by hydrophilic portions protruding into the cytoplasm and the extracellular space. Ion channels can function as allosteric proteins, that is, they exist in two or more conformations: open, closed and, for example, in the case of the sodium channel, inactive.

An idealized diagram of an ion channel is shown in Fig. 19.2. A channel may be considered as a transmembrane protein sitting in the lipid bilayer of the membrane, often anchored to other membrane proteins or to the intracellular cytoskeleton. The macromolecule is generally very large, consisting of several thousand amino acids arranged in one or several polypeptide chains with many hundreds of oligosaccharide chains covalently linked to amino acids on the outer face. When open, the channel forms a water-filled pore extending across the membrane. The pore is much wider than an ion over most of its length and may narrow to atomic dimensions only in a short stretch, the selectivity filter, where the ionic selectivity is established. Hydrophilic amino acids line the pore wall and hydrophobic amino acids line the lipid bilayer. Gating requires a conformational change of the pore

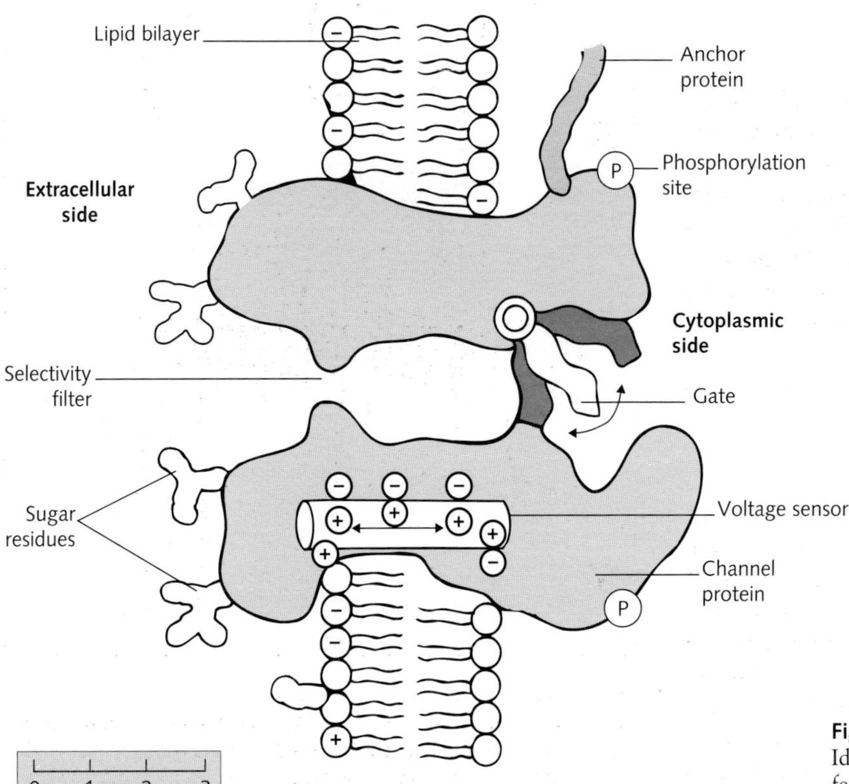

Figure 19.2
Idealized structure of an ion channel. The key features are annotated on the diagram and described fully in the text.

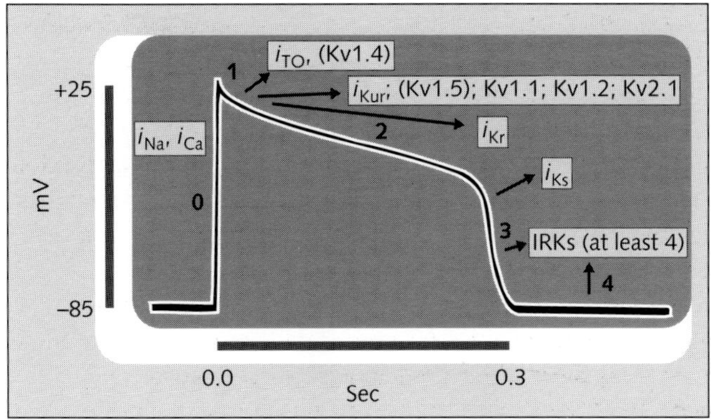

Figure 19.3
K currents of the human cardiac action potential. i_{TO} = the transient outward K current; i_{KUR} = ultrarapidly inactivating delayed rectifying K channel; i_{Kr} and i_{Ks} = rapidly and slowly activating components of i_K the delayed rectifier; IRKs = inwardly rectifying K channels.

that moves a gate into and out of an occluding position. The probabilities of opening and closing are controlled by a sensor. In the case of a voltage-sensitive channel the sensor includes many charged groups that move in the membrane electric field during gating.

19.3 Control of ion-channel activity

In the heart a variety of different types of stimuli controls the activity of ion channels. These include (i) voltage, as in the case of Na^+, Ca^{2+} and K^+ channels; (ii) intracellular second messengers such as cyclic adenosine monophosphate (cAMP) which, for example, regulates the activity of hyperpolarization-activated inward current (i_f) channels of sinoatrial node, and (iii) phosphorylation, which activates or augments the activity of many channels, e.g. Cl^- channels and voltage-activated Ca^{2+} channels.

Ion channels can also be activated by changes in cell volume and membrane tension (Chapter 10).

19.4 Range of channel types

Previous chapters have dealt with the different membrane currents which underlie the cardiac action potential. Many of the individual proteins and genes coding for them have now been identified and characterized in detail at the molecular level. This has led to the identification of many different classes and subtypes of Na^+, Ca^{2+} and K^+ channel and to the recognition of additional subtle differences between the channels of different species and tissues. For example, at least 10 K^+ channel genes encode the plateau and repolarizing phase of the cardiac action potential (Fig. 19.3).

19.4.1 Voltage-gated Na^+ and Ca^{2+} channels

The geometry of ion channels, determined by identifying hydrophilic and hydrophobic regions of the protein structure, is often illustrated using folding diagrams which depict areas of the protein structure (domains) that are cytoplasmic, membrane-spanning and extracellular. The voltage-gated Na^+ and Ca^{2+} channels (Fig. 19.4) found in the heart are constructed from a single large polypeptide chain. The precise way in which this large protein is organized in relation to the membrane is not yet certain but proposed schemes for Na^+ and Ca^{2+} channels are shown in Fig. 19.4a and b.

In the case of both Na^+ and Ca^{2+} channels, the polypeptide includes: (i) four membrane-spanning domains (I–IV); (ii)

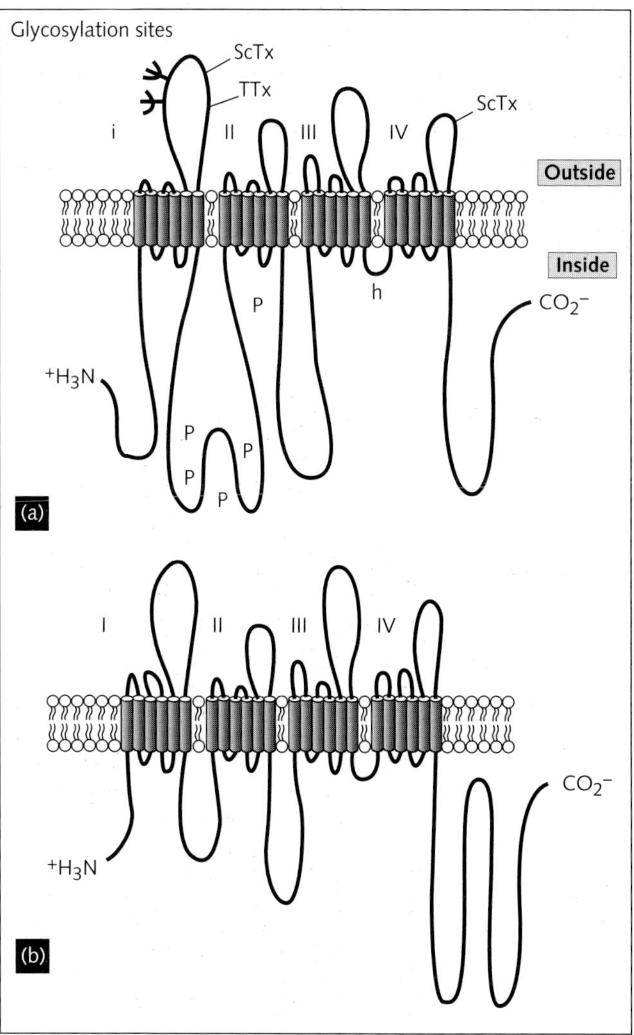

Figure 19.4
Proposed folding diagram of the principal subunits of voltage-gated (a) Na^+ and (b) Ca^{2+} channels. Internal repeats are labelled I–IV. P regions of the peptide chain represent phosphorylation sites. ScTx, TTx: saxitoxin and tetrodotoxin binding sites.

cytoplasmic domains which include amino-terminal and carboxy-terminal ends of the polypeptide chain and long loops linking domains I and II, II and III and III and IV; and (iii) shorter extracellular loops. Domains I–IV are called repeats since they are identical, each consisting of six hydrophobic membrane-spanning regions that probably possess an α-helical structure. Domains I–IV are thought to be arranged in a group of four (a tetramer) to give a central ion channel.

It is on the cytoplasmic loops that sites for phosphorylation are located; fewer amino acid residues are positioned in the extracellular space, the majority coming from the loop between the membrane-spanning regions S5 and S6. In the case of Na^+ channels this region of the polypeptide chain is associated with binding sites for hydrophilic toxins such as the Na^+ channel blocker, tetrodotoxin.

A region of each of the membrane-spanning domains, the S4 region, probably forms the actual voltage sensor. On depolarization this is thought to move within the membrane lipid which leads to opening of the channel pore. The pore itself (known as the P3 region) acts as a selectivity filter.

Some ion channels are made up by the association of more than one type of protein together in a polymeric complex. Calcium channels are an example of this. The four classes of calcium channel (T, L, N and P) known to date can be distinguished by their electrophysiological profile and pharmacology. L-type calcium channels are complexes composed of a pore-forming α_1 subunit and four small accessory proteins α_2, β, γ and δ (Fig. 19.5) which are thought to regulate the behaviour of the channel in response to physiological stimuli.

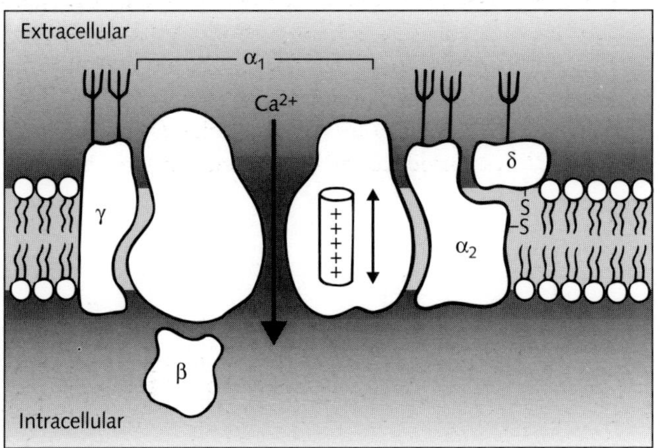

Figure 19.5
Subunits of the L-type Ca^{2+} channel. All subunits except β have some hydrophobic domains and are expected to be membrane-associated. The α_2 and δ peptides are linked by disulphide bonds and are encoded in the same gene. Tridents represent glycosylation sites.

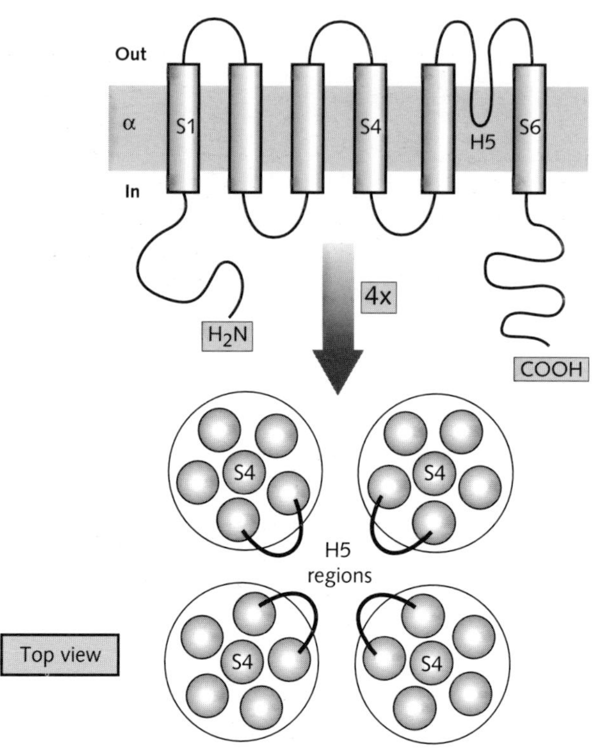

Figure 19.6
Voltage gated (K_V) channels consist of a tetrameric arrangement of the α subunits embedded in the plasma membrane of excitable cells. Each α subunit consists of six membrane-spanning regions with a voltage sensor. Proposed structure of an α subunit is shown above and the tetrameric arrangement of the four α subunits viewed from above is shown below.

19.4.2 Voltage-gated K^+ channels

Voltage-gated K^+ channels, members of the so-called K_V family, are different in structure from the voltage-gated Na^+ and Ca^{2+} channels. They are thought to consist of four separate identical α subunits (Fig. 19.6) which come together to form a channel. These α subunits possess six potential transmembrane domains (S1–S6). The S4 region is believed, like that of the voltage-gated Na^+ and Ca^{2+} channels, to form the voltage sensor. The H5 region, between S5 and S6, much of which forms an extracellular loop, is thought to form the channel pore and to impart ion selectivity. It is the molecular region with the highest degree of amino acid sequence homology in all known K channels. Inactivation of K_V channels is thought to involve a 'ball-and-chain' peptide attached to one or more of the K channel subunits. The ball is positively charged and the charges attract it to its binding site, resulting in channel inactivation. The binding site is thought to be located within the domain that connects the S4 and S5 segments of the channel protein.

19.4.3 Inwardly rectifying K (i_{KI}) channels

The structure of i_{KI} channels is quite different from that of other K channels because each protein contains only two transmembrane domains (M1 and M2) separated by a sequence strongly homologous with the pore (H5) region of other voltage-gated K channels (Fig. 19.7). As in the K_V family, however, i_{KI} channels may also have tetrameric structure since it is thought that four individual protein molecules group together to form a functional channel.

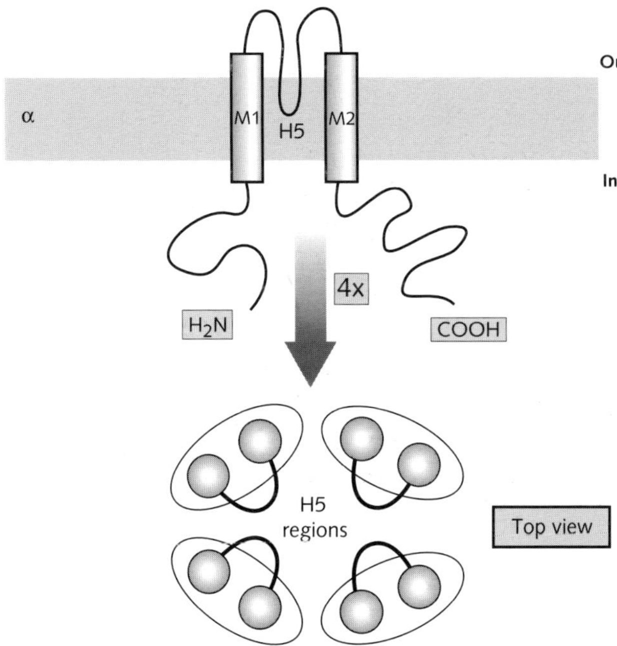

Figure 19.7
Proposed transmembrane looping of the principal subunits of an inwardly rectifying K^+ channel and the proposed tetrameric arrangement in the membrane.

19.4.4 Cl^- channels

The predominant type of Cl^- channel found in the heart is opened by protein kinase A phosphorylation as a consequence of β-adrenoreceptor stimulation. This channel, a 1480-amino-acid protein known as the cystic fibrosis transmembrane regulator (CFTR), is the product of the cystic fibrosis gene. This protein contains two major structural regions, each having six membrane-spanning domains and a cytoplasmic nucleotide-binding domain. Between these two structural regions lies a 240-amino-acid regulatory domain containing several phosphorylation sites (Fig. 19.8).

19.5 Methods used to study ion channels

19.5.1 Patch clamping (see Fig. 4.1)

The aspects of channel function for which each configuration can be used are summarized below:

- *Cell-attached* allows examination of ion-channel modulation by intracellular second messengers such as cAMP or Ca^{2+} in an intact cellular environment.
- *Outside-out* allows examination of channel modulators acting from the extracellular surface via membrane-delimited pathways in well-defined media.
- *Inside-out* as above, but from the intracellular membrane surface.
- *Whole-cell* recording allows measurement of ionic currents and action potentials from whole cells while regulating the ionic environment within the cell.

19.5.2 Cloning and the polymerase chain reaction

Cloning is essentially isolation and amplification (i.e. making many copies) of a small amount of DNA. This is often achieved using the polymerase chain reaction (PCR), an enzyme-catalysed reaction for manufacturing DNA. Specific sequences of synthetic DNA only a few bases long (known as primers) have been found to bind to the genome at desired points and the PCR technique is used to amplify the sequence bracketed (see Fig. 19.9 for more details). It is then possible to use DNA to produce mRNA which can then be injected

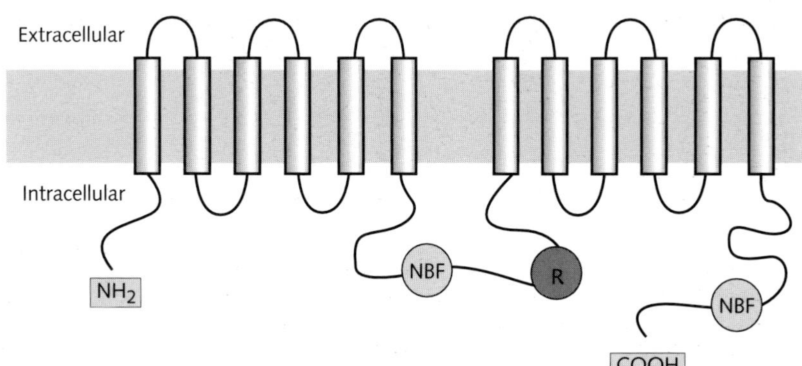

Figure 19.8
The cystic fibrosis transmembrane regulator (CFTR; a Cl^- channel) is thought to consist of 12 transmembrane spanning α helices, two nucleotide-binding folds (NBF) and a regulatory (R) domain.

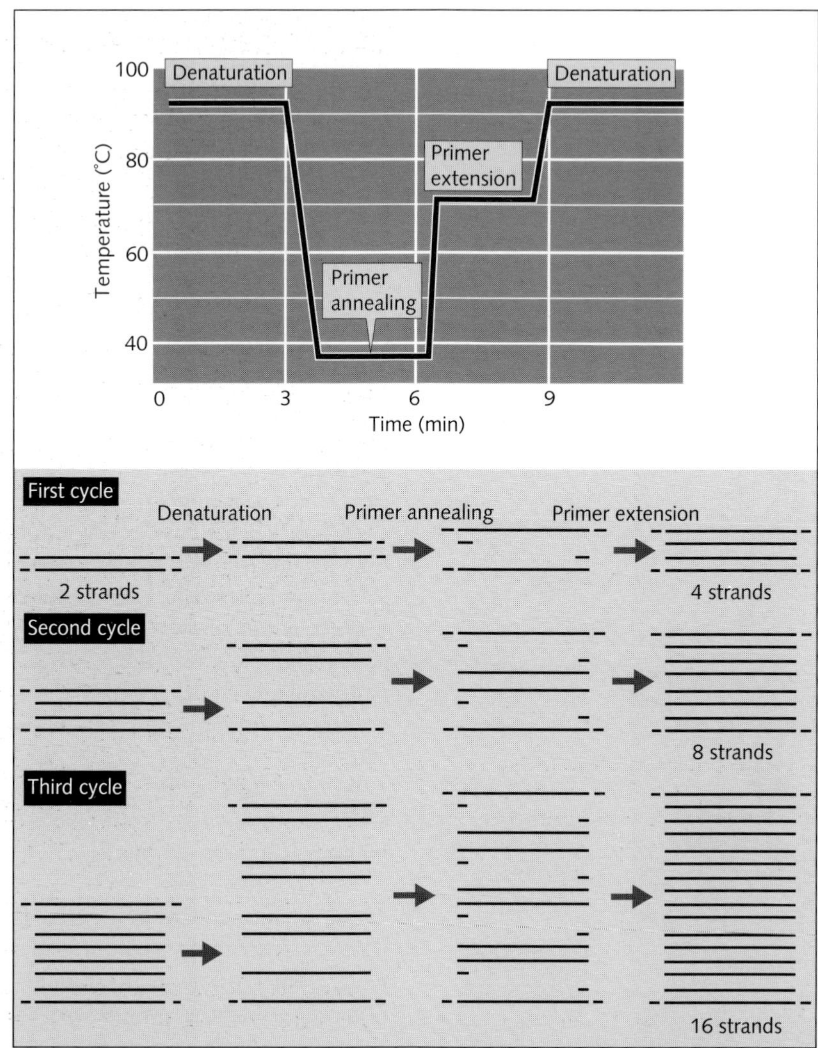

Figure 19.9
The polymerase chain reaction. Two oligonucleotide probes (or primers) are synthesized or isolated. These are added to the sample of DNA to be amplified. The DNA is then heat-*denatured* (at 95°C), resulting in the separation of the strands, and then allowed to cool to 40°C. Under these conditions the primers hybridize or *anneal* with the genomic DNA with their 3′ ends pointing towards each other. Addition of a heat-stable enzyme DNA polymerase (isolated from the thermophilic bacterium *Thermus aquaticus*) and elevation of the temperature to 70°C allows *extension* of these primers from some 50 to 3500 bases. This gives two new double-stranded sections of DNA. Since the extension products of each primer can serve as templates for the other primer, the whole process can be continued in a cyclical manner with each cycle doubling the amount of DNA bracketed by the primers. Amplification is exponential and thus 20–30 cycles can amplify a particular sequence 10^5 or more times. (Three cycles are shown.)

into an expression system such as a toad oocyte or cell-line. Thus a previously inert cell not possessing a particular channel can be made to express it, providing an ideal system for electrophysiological investigation of the channel.

19.5.3 Site-directed mutagenesis

The PCR reaction can be used to produce DNA coding for a particular channel possessing mutations (i.e. with an altered sequence of nucleotide bases). This can then be used to produce correspondingly mutated RNA which can be expressed as described above. Such mutations may involve substitution or deletion of a given amino acid. For example, in the case of inwardly rectifying K channels, substitution of an aspartate for an asparagine in the M2 region turns the channel into one with a linear current–voltage profile (Fig. 19.10), indicating that this amino acid residue plays a major role in regulating the gating of this channel.

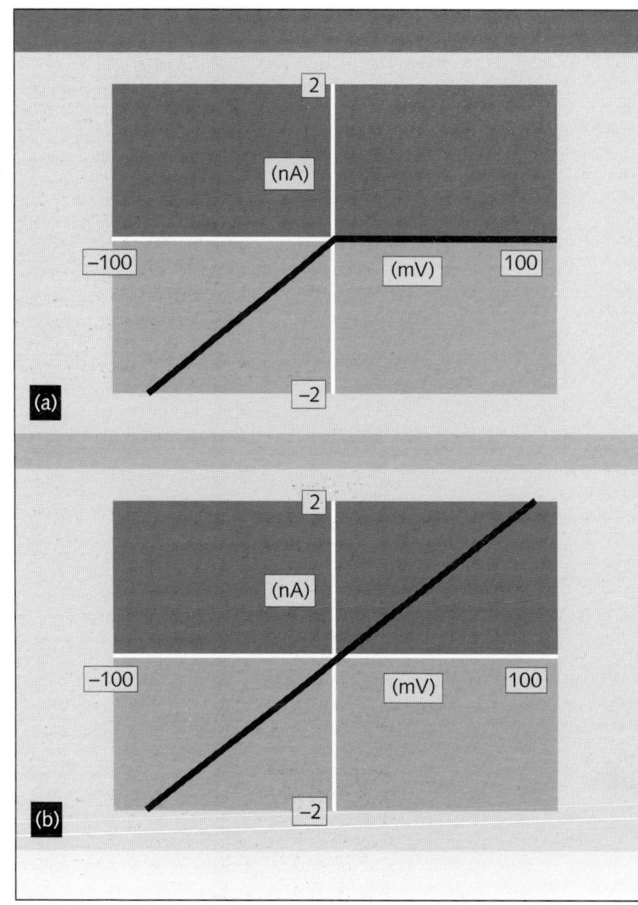

Figure 19.10
Current–voltage relationship for a cardiac inwardly rectifying channel. (a) Note that the channel only passes current in an inward direction (light shading). (b) Following substitution of an aspartate for an asparagine in the M2 region, inward rectification is removed and the channel also passes current in the outward direction (dark shading).

19.5.4 Computer modelling

Channel structures can be modelled on a computer. This involves comparing the amino acid sequences of regions thought to represent the pore and the transmembrane-spanning domains with other proteins known to possess some sequence homology and which have had their structures defined. In the case of the potassium channel, the actual pore region has been modelled in this way. The validity of models can be checked by examining the effect that mutations, carried out as described in section 19.4.3, have on channel behaviour and whether they agree with computer predictions.

20 Growing points in cardiac research

20.1 General comments

We hope this book has provided an introductory overview of cardiac physiology and pharmacology. We have tried not to include information which is too speculative or inconclusive and tried to simplify complex research hypotheses to an accessible level. There is, however, a great deal which remains unknown. The exact mechanism of action of some of the drugs currently used in the clinic is still not entirely understood, so that the use of many agents, for example in the therapy of cardiac arrhythmia, is still empirical.

To counteract this problem, millions of dollars are being invested worldwide to fund research into cardiac disease from a variety of new perspectives, including gene therapy, xenotransplants, computer modelling and epidemiological studies. Results of this research are likely to alter radically how cardiac disease will be treated in the future. This chapter briefly highlights some of the areas currently at the forefront of cardiac research.

20.2 Molecular biology and gene therapy

Recent advances in molecular biology have had, and will continue to have, a major and radical influence on the future therapy of cardiac disease. The use of DNA cloning techniques has also heightened our understanding of how the heart functions at a molecular level. This has improved our appreciation of the heart at a macroscopic and multicellular level. Molecular biology is influencing our understanding of the way drugs work, by allowing scientists to isolate proteins of interest and look closely at how drugs interact with them. Such methods have also allowed assays to be developed in which tens of thousands of compounds can be rapidly tested in the search for new drugs.

Molecular biology has also led to the concept and subsequent development of gene therapy. This is basically a technique where DNA, or the genes themselves, are regarded or used as drugs. To put this simply, if a condition is due to expression of a particular protein, the aim is to eliminate the gene encoding the protein and thereby relieve the condition. Conversely, if a protein is lacking, the aim is to insert the appropriate gene that codes for it. Thus a gene or an appropriate string of DNA can be regarded as a 'magic bullet' for a specific problem.

Gene therapy is being heralded as a medical revolution that will radically change our approach to curing disease. It is, however, controversial, and subject to considerable ethical difficulties. Will the technology be abused, resulting in a *Brave New World* situation? Is it appropriate for doctors to 'play God' by manipulating the human genome? These are important issues and no doubt we will be forced into resolving them.

Gene therapy is potentially beneficial for heart disease since the majority of cardiac conditions are related to the genetic predisposition of the individual. For example, recent evidence suggests that long QT syndrome (an inherited cardiac arrhythmia which can cause abrupt loss of consciousness, seizures and sudden death from ventricular tachycardia) is genetically linked. This syndrome is associated with mutations in a part of the gene coding for the cardiac sodium channel and its inactivation and in a second gene similar to ones that encode the α subunits of potassium channels. A further example where the genetic basis of a cardiac disease is being unravelled is that of familial cardiac hypertrophy, a condition which often leads to premature sudden death in affected individuals. Point mutations in any one of four genes can cause this condition; the location of the mutation is known in approximately 40% of cases.

It is important to remember that most cardiac disease is multifactorial. Thus the genetic make-up of an individual may be a contributing factor, but is unlikely to be the whole cause. It follows therefore that gene therapy is unlikely to represent a radical and total cure in every case.

20.3 Computers and cardiac disease

As the molecular identity of the many cardiac proteins is unravelled and their complex interplay investigated, there has been a parallel interest at the cellular and multicellular level in modelling the mechanical and electrical behaviour of the heart. Detailed and accurate mathematical models of cells and of multicellular networks can be constructed enabling researchers to produce and manipulate computer-generated simulations of cardiac activity. The development of parallel computers has made available enough computing power to generate arrhythmias in network simulations; an example is shown in Fig. 20.1. This is particularly useful since arrhythmias are a manifestation of the malfunction of thousands of cells electrically coupled together and cannot be reproduced experimentally in isolated cells. It is hoped that, in the future,

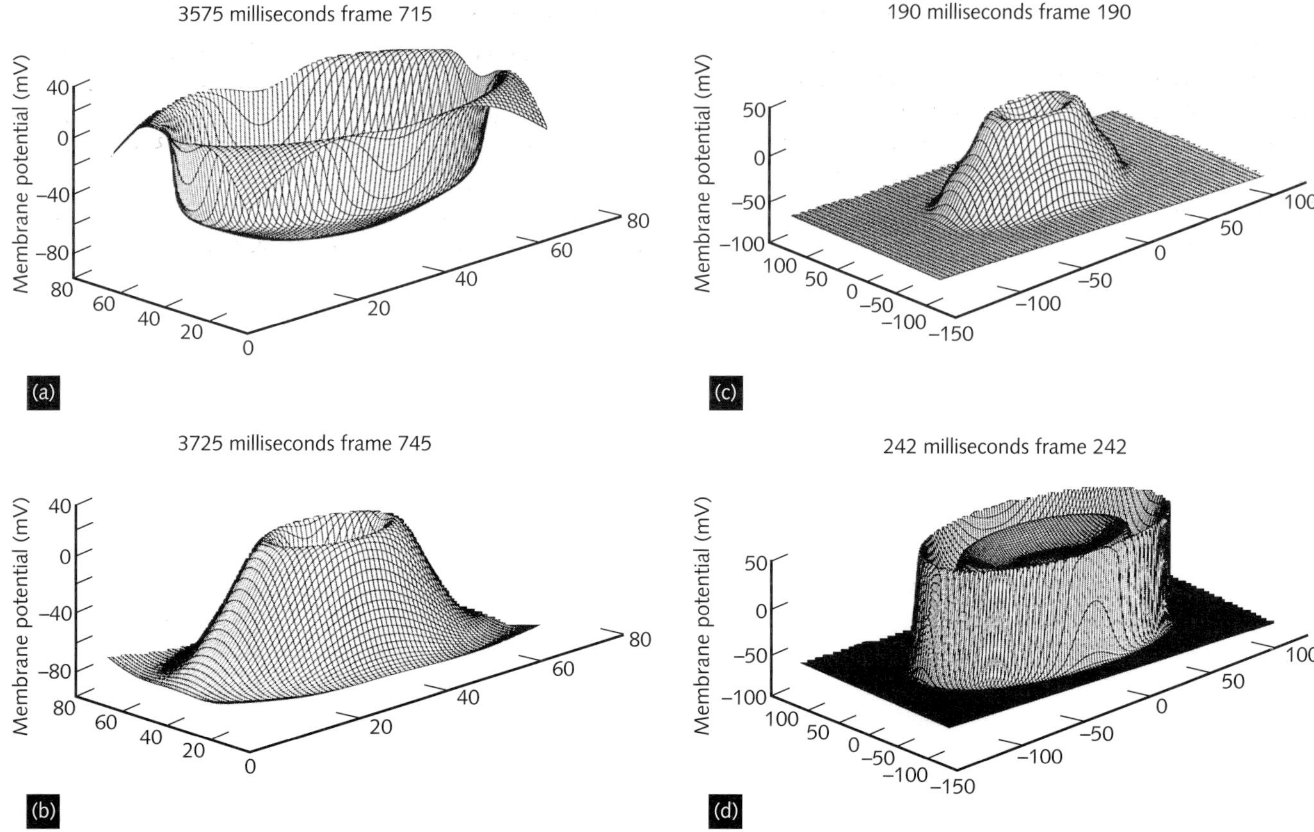

Figure 20.1
Mathematical models of cardiac cell networks created on a parallel computer. (a) Membrane potential in a 128 × 128 sinoatrial node network incorporating regional variation of cell membrane parameters. X- and Y- coordinates represent cell position and the Z-axis encodes membrane potential in mV at time (t) = 3.575 s. Note that firing starts at the periphery of the node. (b) As in (a) with membrane potential displayed at t = 3.725 s. (c) and (d) Pacemaking and conduction in a combined model of the SA node and atrium. A circular SA node with a radius of 63 cells is embedded in a 256 × 256 mesh of surrounding atrial cells. SA node firing is now the normal 'centre first' pattern. Coupling between cells is uniform throughout at 100 nS. (c) shows activation of the SA node at t = 190 ms. (d) Shows propagation of the excitatory impulse within the atrium at t ≈ 242 ms. (Courtesy of Dr R.L. Winslow.)

models of the electrical activity of the heart will allow cardiologists and scientists to predict the best type of drug to use for a given cardiac condition, in addition to allowing them to assess the effects of new drugs.

Increases in the power of computers and their ability to store large quantities of data have also allowed substantial databases to be produced. Such technology can be used to amass a vast amount of epidemiological information which allows population trends and predisposing factors for cardiac disease to be monitored and related to incidence.

20.4 Xenotransplantation

In 1995 approximately 6000 patients in the UK were waiting for organs — 1000 of these for hearts — with the number growing at 5% per annum. Despite the need for long-term treatment with immunosuppressant drugs, heart transplantation has been very successful, with 77% of hearts still functioning after 5 years. Organs suitable for transplantation are difficult to find owing to our ageing population, improved road safety and lack of intensive care facilities. Thus surgeons have been looking for alternatives to human organs for transplantation. Xenotransplantation (the use of animal organs) represents a potential alternative. The major problem with xenotransplants is the phenomenon of immediate rejection. One approach to this problem is to use organs from genetically modified animals, particularly pigs. Transgenic pigs possess organs which are less susceptible to rejection since some of the animal genes central to the rejection process have been replaced with human ones. Preliminary experiments with monkeys transplanted with transgenic pig hearts have proved very promising, and may pave the way for the transplantation of pig hearts into humans.

The major problem that may be associated with successful

xenotransplantation is the possible emergence of a new virulent disease which might cross the species barrier to humans with the transplanted tissue. Other problems relate to the interaction of the xenotransplant with other body systems. Will the host's hormones affect the transplant in the same manner as the original organ? Finally, there may be objections on religious and ethical grounds to such transplantation.

20.5 Conclusion

With the advent of all these new and exciting technologies, the future holds considerable promise for the therapy of cardiac disease. Although it is likely that in the short to medium term traditional drug therapy will still predominate, a book (or its digital successor) covering similar ground to this one in the second quarter of the next century will probably describe radically different treatments.

O | Further reading

Aidley, D.J. (1989) *The Physiology of Excitable Cells*, 3rd edn. Cambridge University Press, Cambridge.

Akhtar, M., Breithart, G., Camm, A.J. *et al.* (1990) CAST and beyond: implications of the cardiac arrhythmia suppression trial. *Circulation* **81**, 1123–1127.

Bray, J.J. *et al.* (1994) *Lecture Notes on Human Physiology*, 3rd edn. Blackwell Scientific Publications, Oxford.

Camm, A.J. (ed.). (1993) *Arrhythmia Octet.* (Eight review papers from the *Lancet.*)

CAST (1989) The Cardiac Arrhythmias Suppression Trial investigators. Preliminary report: effect of encainide and flecainide on mortality in a randomized trial of arrhythmia suppression after myocardial infarction. *New England Journal of Medicine* **321**, 406–412.

Eisner, D.A. & Trafford, A.W. (1996) A sideways look at sparks, quarks, puffs and blips. *Journal of Physiology* **497**, 2.

Fozzard, H.A., Haber, E., Jennings, R.B., Katz, A.M. & Morgan, H.E. (eds) (1986) *The Heart and Cardiovascular System. Scientific Foundations*. Raven Press, New York.

Hardman, J.G. *et al.* (eds) (1996) *Goodman and Gilman's The Pharmacological Basis of Therapeutics*, 9th edn. McGraw Hill, New York.

Hille, B. (1992) *Ionic Channels of Excitable Membranes*, 2nd edn. Sinauer Associates Inc., Sunderland MA.

Irisawa, H., Brown H.F. & Giles W. (1993) Pacemaking in the sinoatrial node. *Physiological Reviews*, **72**, 391–410.

Keech, A., Collins, R., MacMahon, S. *et al.* (1994) Three-year follow-up of the Oxford Cholesterol Study: assessment of the efficacy and safety of simvastin in preparation for a large mortality study. *European Heart Journal* **15**, 255–269.

Levick, J.R. (1995) *An Introduction to Cardiovascular Physiology*, 2nd edn. Butterworth Heinemann, London.

Marmot, M.G. *et al.* (1994) *Nutritional Aspects of Cardiovascular Disease.* Department of Health Committee on Medical Aspects of Food Policy Cardiovascular Review Group. HMSO.

Morad, M., Ebashi, S., Trautwein, W. & Kurachi, Y. (eds) (1996) *Molecular Physiology and Pharmacology of Cardiac Ion Channels.* Kluwer, Dordrecht.

Mubagwa, K., Mullane, K. & Flameng, W. (1996) Role of adenosine in the heart and circulation. *Circulation Research* **32**, 797–813.

Noble, D. (1979) *The Initiation of the Heartbeat*, 2nd edn. Oxford University Press, Oxford.

Opie, L.H. (1991) *The Heart. Physiology and Metabolism*, 2nd edn. Raven Press, New York.

Opie, L.H. (1995) *Drugs for the Heart*, 4th edn. WB Saunders Co., Philadelphia.

Rang, H.P. & Dale, M.M. (1995) *Pharmacology*, 3rd edn. Churchill Livingstone, Edinburgh.

Rees, S. & Curtis, M.J. (1996) Which cardiac potassium channel subtype is the preferable channel for suppression of ventricular arrhythmias? *Pharmacology and Therapeutics*, **69**, 199–217.

Taglialatela, M. & Brown, A.M. (1994) Structural correlates of K^+ channel function. *News in Physiological Sciences*, **9**, 169–173.

Timmis, A.D. & Nathan, A.W. (1996) *Essentials of Cardiology*, 3rd edn. Blackwell Science, Oxford.

Vaughan Williams, E.M. (1984) A classification of antiarrhythmic actions reassessed after a decade of new drugs. *Journal of Clinical Pharmacology* **24**, 129–147.

Waldo, A.L., Camm, A.J., de Ruyter, H. *et al.* (1995) SWORD Investigators: preliminary results from the survival with oral D-sotalol (SWORD) trial. *Journal of the American College of Cardiology* **15A**.

Zipes, D.P. & Jalife, J. (1995) *Cardiac Electrophysiology: From Cell to Bedside*, 2nd edn. W.B. Saunders Co., Philadelphia.

O | Index

acebutolol 95
ACE inhibitors 100, 104–5
acetylcholine, effect on heart rate 71–2
acidosis 82–3
actin filaments, muscle contraction 61, 62
adenosine 48–9
adenosine triphosphate-sensitive, potassium channels 41–2
adrenaline 72, 76, 81–2
after-depolarizations 40–1
aldosterone 107–8
alinidine 48–50
α-adrenoceptors 94
amiloride 107–8
amiodarone 47
amrinone 103–4
angina pectoris 88
  complications 90
  treatment 88–9
angiotensin II 105–6
angiotensin-converting enzyme (ACE) inhibitors 100, 104–5
antiarrhythmic drugs 43–51
  class I 43–4, 45
  class II 44–6
  class III 46–7
  class IV 47–8
  'class V' 48–50
  classification 43
  clinical trials 50–1
arrhythmias
  cardiac failure, treatment 100–1
  classification 54
  clinical considerations 53–60
  development 38–42
  electrophysiological basis 37–42
  factors initiating 53
  maintenance 53–4
  pathological consequences 54
  predisposing factors 53
artificial pacemakers 28–9
aspirin, prevention of thrombus formation 94–7
  coronary heart disease 87
atenolol 46, 94–5
ATP sensitive potassium channels 41–2
atrial cells 20–1
atrial fibrillation 55, 56
  electrophysiological basis 37–8
  myocardial infarction 90
atrial flutter 55, 56
  electrophysiological basis 37
atrial tachycardia 54–6
atrioventricular (AV) block 59–60
atrioventricular (AV) nodal re-entrant tachycardia 56–7
atrioventricular (AV) node 13, 26–8
  damage 37
atrioventricular (AV) valves 1
atrium
  conduction pathways 26
  electrical activity 21
autonomic balance 74
  effects of training 77
  in exercise 77
  in heart disease 74–5
autonomic tone 74

Bainbridge reflex 65
bendrofluazide 107, 108
β-adrenoceptors 76, 77, 94
β-blockers 44–6, 94–5
β-sympathomimetic agents 103
blood flow to heart muscles 85
bradyarrhythmias 59–60
bumetanide 107, 108
bundle of His 27

calcium antagonists 47–8
  as antiarrhymics 47–8
  in cardiac failure 106–7
  in ischaemic heart disease 91–3
calcium currents 20–1, 23–4
calcium ion channels 111–12
calcium ions, effects of alterations on heart 81
calcium-release channel, sarcoplasmic reticulum 64–5
calcium sparks 64
captopril 105–6
Cardiac Arrhythmias Suppression Trial (CAST) 44, 50–1
cardiac catheterization 10
cardiac cells, mechanical activation 65
cardiac cycle, mechanical events during 7–10
cardiac failure *see* heart failure
cardiac force, control 72–3
cardiac glycosides 48, 49, 100, 103, 105
cardiac ion channels, structure 109–15
cardiac output measurement 79–80
cardiomyopathy 53, 99–100
  inherited 53
cardioplegic solutions 83
catecholamines
  in arrhythmias 41–2
  catecholamine-induced chloride current 73
  contractility 73
  control of cardiac force 72–3
  heart rate control 71
  receptors 94
chloride channels 66
chloride current, catecholamine-induced 73
chlorothiazide 107, 108
cholesterol 86–7
cholesterol-lowering drugs 87, 94
cholestyramine 94, 96
chordae tendinae 1
circulation
  changes at birth 3
  fetal 2–3, 4
clofibrate 94, 96
cloning, ion channels 113–14
computer modelling, ion channels 115
computers and cardiac disease 117–18
connexin 11
coronary artery bypass graft surgery (CABG) 89
coronary artery disease 53, 85–9
  cardiac failure 99

coronary heart disease 85–7
clinical syndromes 88
prevention 87
risk factors 86–7
coronary vessels 2
control 85
flow through 85
cyclooxygenase 96–7
cystic fibrosis transmembrane regulator 113

defibrillation 59
delayed after-depolarizations 40
delayed rectifier potassium current (i_K) 24, 27
diabetes mellitus, coronary heart disease 87
diastolic depolarization *see* pacemaker depolarization
dichrotic notch 7
diet, coronary heart disease 87
digoxin 48–9, 103–4
dilated cardiomyopathy 99–100
diltiazem 47–8, 91, 93
dipole 33
disopyramide 43, 45
diuretics, cardiac failure 100, 107–8
dobutamine 103–4
dopamine 103–4
Doppler echocardiography 10
ductus arteriosus, closure 3
dye dilution experiment to measure cardiac output 79–80

early after-depolarizations 40–1
echocardiography 9–10
in cardiac failure 100
ectopic beats 54
electrophysiological basis 37
Einthoven
and string galvanometer 15
triangle 33
electrical activity, recording methods 15–16
electrocardiogram 7, 15
electrical dipole 33
electrical vector 33
general electrical features 31–3
in altered potassium 81–2
in arrythmias 55, 57
in diagnosis 33–5
results 33–5
recording 33
enalapril 105–6
encainide 44, 45
equilibrium potentials 19
excitation, conduction 12–13
excitation-contraction coupling 61–5
role of Ca^{2+} ions 61
sequence of events 64
excitatory pathway 11–13
exercise, autonomic balance 75–7
extrasystoles 54

familial cardiac hypertrophy 117
fenofibrate 94
fetal circulation 2–3, 4
fibrillation, electrophysiological basis 37–8
fibroblasts, stretch-sensing 66
flecainide 44, 45
foramen ovale, closure 3
Frank–Starling mechanism 68–9
frusemide 107, 108

gap junctions 11
gemfibrozil 94, 96
gene therapy 117
glyceryl trinitrate 91
G-protein 71, 74, 76
Goldman equation 19

heart
altered ion concentrations, effects on 81–3
block, electrophysiological basis 37–8
congenital malformations 3–5
functional anatomy 1–6
monitoring performance 7–10
sounds 7–8
heart failure
causes 99–100
diagnosis 100
epidemiology 99
myocardial infarction 90
prognosis 101
symptoms 100
transplants 101
treatment 100–1
drugs 103–8
heart rate, control
parasympathetic 71–2
sympathetic 71
heartbeat, changes in pressure during 7
heterometric regulation 68–9
high density lipoprotein (HDL) 87, 94
homeometric regulation 72–3
hydralazine 106, 107
hyperkalaemia, re-entry in 39–40
hyperlipidaemia, coronary heart disease 87
hyperpolarization-activated inward current (i_f) 23, 26
hypertension
coronary heart disease 86
heart failure 99
hypertrophic cardiomyopathy 100
hypoxia, arrhythmias 41–2

$i_{b,Na}$ (inward background current) 24, 27
$i_{Ca,L}$ (L-type calcium current) 20–3, 46, 48, 71
$i_{Ca,T}$ (T-type calcium current) 24
i_f (hyperpolarization-activated inward current) 23, 26, 49
i_K (delayed rectifier potassium current) 21, 24
i_{K1} (inward rectifier potassium current) 21, 47
$i_{K,ACh}$ (acetylcholine-induced potassium current) 71
$i_{K,ATP}$ (ATP-sensitive potassium channels) 41
i_{Na} (inward sodium current) 19, 45
$i_{Na,Ca}$ (sodium calcium exchange current) 18, 21
i_{to} (transient outward current) 21, 47
implantable cardioverter defibrillator (ICD) 58, 59
inotropic drugs, cardiac failure 100, 103
intercellular connections 11
inward background current 24, 27
inward rectifier potassium channel (i_{K1}) 21, 47
ion channels
control of activity 111
formation 110
methods used to study 113–15
molecular biology 109–15
structure 110–12
types 111–13
ion-channel protein, synthesis 109
ischaemic heart disease, drug treatment 91–8
isosorbide dinitrate 91
cardiac failure 106, 107

jugular venous pulse 8–9

Keith and Flack 12
Kolliker and Müller 15

labetalol 95
law of Laplace 69–70
left-to-right shunts 4
length-tension curve 67–8
lignocaine 43
long QT syndrome 53, 117
loop diuretics 107–8
lovastatin 94, 96
low density lipoprotein (LDL) 85, 94

magnetic resonance imaging 10
maximum diastolic potential (SA node cell) 23
mechanoelectric feedback 65–6
membrane current mechanisms 17–18
membrane potential 19
metoprolol 44, 46, 94–5
mexiletine 43, 45
milrinone 103–4
mitral valve 1
M-mode echocardiography 10
molecular biology
  cardiac ion channels 109–15
  and heart disease 117
muscle, heart
  blood flow 85
  contraction, functional aspects 67–70
  detection of damage 33–5
  function, graphical representation 67
  intracellular membranous system 61–4
myocardial infarction 88
  complications 90
  treatment 90
myocardial ischaemia 87–9
myofilaments, sensitivity to pCa 88
myosin filaments, muscle contraction 61, 62

Na^+/Ca^+ exchange 18
Na^+-K^+ ATPase (Na/K pump) 18, 103
nadolol 95
negative inotropic effect 73
Nernst equation 19
nexi 11
nicardipine 91, 93
nicorandil 92, 94
nicotinic acid 94, 96
nifedipine 47, 91, 93
nimodipine 91, 93
nitrates 91
  cardiac failure 106
Noma, A. 41
nuclear cardiology 10

obesity, coronary heart disease 87
output, cardiac, measurement 79–80

P wave 32
pacemaker depolarization 23–4, 27
pacemaker region 11–12
pacemakers, artificial 28–9
pacemaking
  Purkinje fibres 28–9
  sinoatrial node cells 23–5, 27
papillary muscles 1
parasympathetic supply to heart
  heart rate 71
  negative inotropic effect 73
patch clamping, ion channels 15–16, 113
patent ductus arteriosus 4
percutaneous transluminal coronary angioplasty (PTCA) 89
pH control 82–3
phophodiesterase (PDE) inhibitors 103
pindolol 95
plaque formation 85–6
polymerase chain reaction 113–14
positive inotropic effect 72–3
  cellular basis 73
potassium, effect of alterations on heart 81–2
potassium channel openers 92–4
potassium channels 112–13
  ATP-sensitive 41–2
  delayed rectifier (i_K) channels 21, 24, 27, 47
  drugs blocking 46–7
  inward rectifier (i_{K1}) channels 21, 47
  K_{ACh} channels 71
  structure 112–13
potassium-sparing diuretics 107–8
procainamide 43, 45
propranolol 46, 95
prostacyclin 96–7
Purkinje fibres 13
  location and arrangement 27
  pacemaking 28–9

QRS complex 32
quinidine 43
quinine 45

recording methods 16
re-entry 38–40
  tachyarrhythmias 56–8
refractory period 17, 18
renin 104–5
resting membrane potential 19
restrictive cardiomyopathy 100
right heart, pressure changes 7
right-to-left shunts 4–5
ryanodine receptors 63–4

sarcoplasmic reticulum 63–4
  calcium-release channel 64–8
semilunar valves 2
sick sinus syndrome 59
simvastatin 94
sinoatrial node 12, 13, 23
  cells
    maximum diastolic potential 23
    pacemaking 23–6
sinoatrial pacemaking mechanism 27
sinus bradycardia 59
site-directed mutagenesis, ion channels 114
smoking, coronary heart disease 86
smooth muscle, vascular 92–4
sodium calcium exchange
  in action of digoxin 103
  in action potential 21
  in arrthymias 40
sodium channels, drugs blocking 43–4
sodium current 19–20
sodium ion channels 111–12
sodium ions, effects of alterations on heart 82
sodium nitroprusside 106–7
sodium pump *see* Na^+-K^+ATPase
sotalol 47
spironolactone 107–8
ST segment, myocardial damage 34–5, 90
Starling curve 68
  shift by catecholamines 75
Starling's law of the heart 68–9
  cellular basis 69
stenosis 5
Stokes–Adams attack 59
streptokinase 97–8
stretch-activated channels 65–6

stroke volume
  effect of catecholamines 72–3
  extrinsic regulation 72
  intrinsic control 68–9
supraventricular tachyarrhythmias 54–6
survival with oral *d*-sotalol (SWORD) trial 47
sympathetic nervous system activation, arrhythmias 53

T wave 32
  in hyperkalaemia 81–2
  in hypokalaemia 82
Tawara, S. 12
terminal cisternae 63–4
tetralogy of Fallot 4–5
thermal dilution method, for cardiac output measurement 80
thiazide diuretics 107–8
thrombolytic drugs 98
thromboxane A_2 96–7
thrombus formation 85–6
  preventive action of aspirin 94–6
tissue plasminogen activator (t-PA) 98
tocainide 43, 45
torsade de pointes 41, 53, 59
training, autonomic balance 77
transplantation, cardiac failure 101
tricuspid valve 1
troponin C 69
T-tubules 61–4
two-dimensional echocardiography 10

valves 1–2
valvular heart disease 99
vasodilators 91–4
  cardiac failure 100, 103–7
ventricular arrhythmias, myocardial infarction 90
ventricular cell 15
  action potential 15–17
    membrane currents underlying 17–19
    plateau 20–1
    repolarization 21
    upstroke 19–20
  refractory period 17
  resting (diastolic) potential 19
ventricular fibrillation 59
  electrophysiological basis 37–8
ventricular premature beat 18, 53
ventricular tachyarrhythmias 58–9
ventricular tachycardia
  electrophysiological basis 37–8
  non-sustained 58
  sustained monomorphic 58–9
verapamil 47–8, 91, 93
very low density lipoprotein (LDL) 94
voltage clamping 15

Waller, A.D. 31
Watson and Crick 109
Wenkebach 43
Wenkebach heart block 38
Wolff–Parkinson–White syndrome 40, 53, 54, 57–8
work of the heart xi

xenotransplantation, 118

zatebradine 49–50